When the World Falls Apart

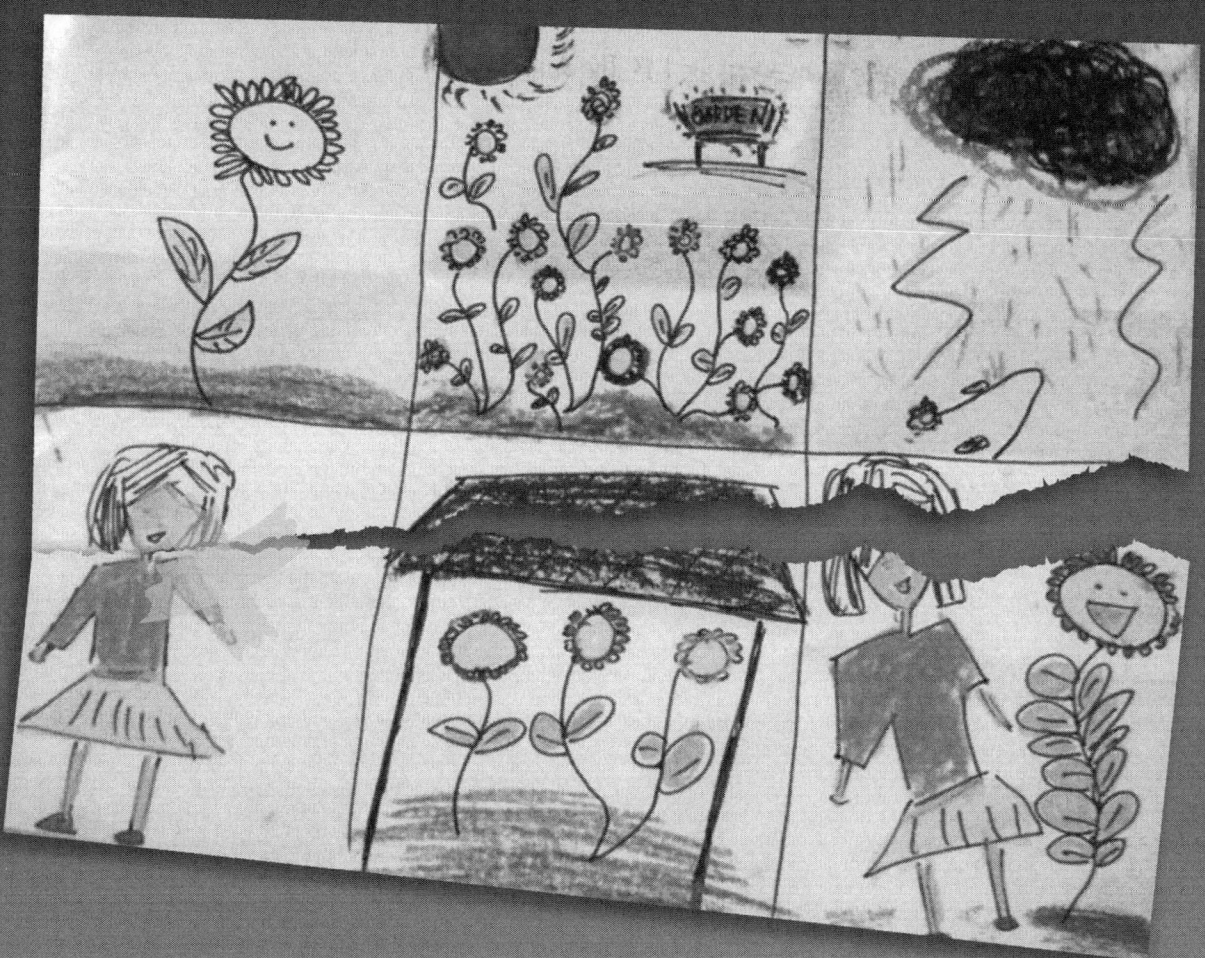

When the World Falls Apart

Working with the Effects of Trauma

SUE JENNINGS

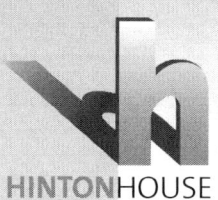

This book is dedicated with love, respect and affection to Professor Mooli Lahad, who inspired and supported me with my trauma work

Thank you Charlie Meyer for the inspirational monster pictures.

Matyas Fazakis created the worksheets and diagrams.

First published in 2015 by

Hinton House Publishers Ltd, Newman House, 4 High Street, Buckingham, MK18 1NT, UK
T +44 (0)1280 822557   F +44 (0) 560 3135274   E info@hintonpublishers.com

www.hintonpublishers.com

© 2015 Sue Jennings

All rights reserved. The whole of this work including texts and illustrations is protected by copyright. No part of it may be copied, altered, adapted or otherwise exploited in any way without express prior permission, except in accordance with the provisions of the Copyright, Designs and Patents Act 1988 or in order to photocopy or make duplicating masters of those pages so indicated, without alteration and including copyright notices, for the express purpose of instruction and examination. No parts of this work may otherwise be loaded, stored, manipulated, reproduced, or transmitted in any form or by any means, electronic or mechanical, including photocopying or storing it in any information, storage or retrieval system, without prior written permission from the publisher, on behalf of the copyright owner.

British Library Cataloguing in Publication Data
A CIP catalogue record for this book is available from the British Library.

ISBN 978 1 906531638

Printed and bound in the United Kingdom by Hobbs the Printers Ltd

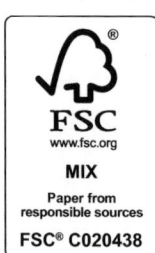

Contents

List of Worksheets — vii

List of Story Sheets — ix

Acknowledgments — xi

About the Author — xiii

Foreword *Professor Mooli Lahad* — xv

Section One: Introduction — 1

Section Two: The Building Blocks of Recovery: the Body & the Brain — 7

Section Three: Identifying Coping Strengths in Children & Young People who have Experienced Trauma: Using the Six-Part Story Approach — 17

Section Four: Self-Soothing & Self-Care — 37

Section Five: The Safe Place — 49

Section Six: Night Fears & Nightmares — 61

Section Seven: Challenging the Monsters — 73

Section Eight: Trees — 93

Section Nine: Healing Stories	105
Resources	131
Group Contract & Agreement	132
Additional Healing Stories	
1 The Transformation of Sedna	133
2 The Story of the Brave Little Goat: Why the Tapir Has No Tail	135
3 The Children of Wax: a Story from Africa	138
Certificate of Achievement	140
Warm Up & Drama Games	141
References & Further Reading	147
Information on Training	149

Worksheets

3a	Story in Six Parts	32
3b	Story Circle or Mandala	33
3c	Circles of Protection: Personal	34
3d	Circles of Protection: Social	35
3e	Chains of Qualities and Strengths	36
4a	Hand Massage	44
4b	Special Scents & Smells	45
4c	Pleasant & Soothing Touch	46
4d	Special Food & Taste	47
4e	Special Sounds	48
5a	Where do I Feel Safe?	55
5b	Where do I Not Feel Safe?	56
5c	Safe Pictures in My Head	57
5d	Scary Pictures in My Head	58
5e	Creating a Safe Place	59
6a	When it Gets Dark ... the Scary Moments	67
6b	When it Gets Dark ... the Good Moments	68
6c	How Can Other People Help?	69
6d	How Can I Help Myself?	70
6e	Waking Up Nightmares	71

7a	Monsters in the Shadows	79
7b	How I Feel Inside	80
7c	Challenging the Monster	81
7d	Scary Spaces & Places	82
7e	Talking to the Dream Monster	83
7f	The Story of My Monster	84
7g	Scary Shadows	86
7h	The Monster Under the Bed	88
7i	Meeting & Welcoming the Monster	90
8a	Falling Leaves	99
8b	Learning to Play	100
8c	Shelters in the Tree	101
8d	Climbing Trees Again	102
8e	Tree of Friends	103
9a	David and Goliath 1	125
9b	David and Goliath 2	126
9c	The Flowering Tree	127
9d	The Story of the Brave Little Goat 1	128
9e	The Story of the Brave Little Goat 2	129

Story Sheets

Story 1   The Magic Bag: a Roma Story from Hungary   112

Story 2   Saint Peter & the Wolves: a traditional story from Romania   115

Story 3   How Coyote Helped the Karok People to Get Fire: a Native
           American Story   118

Story 4   The Flowering Tree: a Tale from South India   120

Story 5   The Hero's Journey   124

Additional Story 1   The Transformation of Sedna (an Inuit Story)   133

Additional Story 2   The Story of Little Goat: Why the Tapir
                      has no Tail (a Malay Story)   135

Additional Story 3   The Children of Wax: a Story from Africa   138

Acknowledgements

Dr Lai Fong Hwa, Indranee Liew and Priscilla Ho, as well as colleagues and students in Malaysia have been a source of strength and support. My colleagues and friends in Romania, especially those involved with the projects with the homeless teenagers, have been a constant source of creativity and friendship.

My appreciation also goes to Lemsip and my bank manager who have sustained me during this writing period!

Thank you Sarah Miles for being a great and supportive publisher!

Sue Jennings
Stratford-upon-Avon, Warwickshire
Zarnesti, Transylvania

About the Author

Sue Jennings PhD is Honorary Fellow at Leeds Metropolitan University and Visiting Professor, Taiwan National University of the Arts. She has been a pioneering influence in the development of dramatherapy in several countries, and has established Neuro-Dramatic-Play as an approach to attachment that emphasises the importance of early playfulness. She has written numerous books, many of them translated into Greek, Korean, Russian, Swedish, Danish and Italian. Her doctoral research was carried out with the Temiar people in the Malaysian rainforest, where she lived with her three children. Currently she works through play with children and teenagers in Romania and trains carers in 'Creative Care' in their work with older people and people with dementia. She was awarded a Churchill Fellowship for Arts and Older People, 2012–2013.

www.suejennings.com
www.creativecareinternational.org

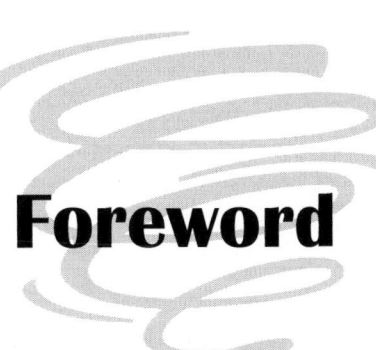

Foreword

Trauma and the Contribution of Neuro-Dramatic-Play and Fairy Stories

Mooli Lahad

The book in your hand is a treasure of knowledge wisdom and skills. It encompasses up-to-date research as well as wisdom beyond time.

When we talk about children I have found that exploring the world of fairy tales is a never-ending path to make sense for us and for them, of what this world is about, or as Sue Jennings calls it 'Making sense of the world around us'.

It is amazing to see how Neuro-Dramatic-Play appears in these stories, and how arousal and 'Fight, Flight and Freeze' also takes place in them. It is unclear why so many of the stories for children and those that were 'assigned' to them (fairy tales) are so cruel and full of trauma, pain and sorrow. Is this the traditional way to reactivate neurons in thebrain so that trauma will be acknowledged, related to, desensitized and then recovered from, througpositive endings?

One of the most interesting fairy tales addressing a Neuro-Dramatic impasse is the story of Little Red Riding Hood. There are many aspects that can be explored in the story, such as the relations with her mother, who knows about wolves, but does not prepare her daughter for this encounter. Why did she send a little girl all by herself through the forest?

But before going any further into the story let's take a moment to ask ourselves some important questions about Little Red Riding Hood. Prior to the encounter at Granny's house, did she know Granny at all? Did she know the wolf before the encounter at Granny's house? If the answers to the above questions are yes, ask yourself: how old is 'Little Red Riding Hood'? Would you agree that she is not 5–7 years? So, why in the most remembered part of the story, the moment where she opens the door and sees: 'There lay her grandmother with her cap pulled far over her face, and looking very strange.' Why is she not running away?

Foreword

Why is she stating the three big statements:

◆ Grandma, what big ears you have ...

◆ What big eyes you have ...

◆ What big teeth you have ...

Because a child in trouble, a little girl who is given a too big task for her age and capability, who feels trapped, does not therefore, believe in her own senses. The trauma of feeling entrapped with the aggressor, the fear of what has happened to Granny, triggers the frightened amygdala part of the brain to fire 'Freeze'. More and more Freeze, and the hippocampus learns to interpret any sign as a threat, a danger, and does not allow the brain to judge: is it a real threat? Is it a neutral sign or is it a loving and caring sign?

Therapeutic play, drama and storytelling, is very much about developing the child's confidence in her own senses. Believing in what she feels, expressing it and feeling safe in so doing. By being able to believe in her own senses, she regains control over her life and authenticity; the way in which she relates to the world and others. And that is a very difficult task! And it is one of the tasks that this book strives to teach therapists and teachers as well as parents.

How do we reintroduce the ability to trust one own senses? Are we being overprotective? Directive? Passive?

In order to address this issue in a metaphoric way, allow me to share with you a beautiful Buddhist story.

> *This is the story of a small child who came to his teacher, the Guru. The Guru was holding something in his hand which the child did not recognize and so he asked him what it was. The Guru said 'this is a cocoon, and inside it, lays a beautiful butterfly, soon the cocoon will open and the butterfly will come out.'*
>
> *'Can I have it' asked the child? 'Yes' said the Guru 'but on one condition, that when the cocoon opens and the butterfly comes flapping with his wings to get out, you will not help it. You should not assist it by breaking the shell. The butterfly must do it on its own.'*
>
> *The child promises and took the cocoon and went home. For hours he watched the cocoon until he saw some movements inside, the cocoon moved and slowly there was a little crack and a beautiful fragile little butterfly was flapping its wings so slowly and so weak that it looked it will never be able to come out.*

The little boy watched it and felt he ought to help. Suddenly, despite the Guru's instructions, he broke the cocoon in half and let the butterfly out. The beautiful butterfly started to fly waving his wings for a while but soon it fell on the ground motionless.

The boy picked it up and looked at the dead butterfly, he was crying as he was sadly walking to the Guru's house holding it in his hands.

Showing the dead butterfly, the Guru said: 'you see son, you cracked the cocoon for it, didn't you?' 'Yes, said the boy. 'Well' said the old man, 'you are not to blame; you didn't know that when the butterfly gets out of the cocoon, its only way to strengthen its wings is by flapping them toward the cocoon. It hits and hits its wings until the muscles get strong enough for it to fly; by helping it and breaking the cocoon too soon you prevented it from strengthening its wings and that is why it fell dead ...'

And that is our very delicate role in therapy; we ought to be there, to be present and supportive but not be tempted to do the job: the important job of growing strong muscles for our young clients. It is difficult, it takes time; it is a mixture of patience, experience, exploration and trust.

This book is about this delicate balance between protection and support, guidance and security, knowledge and experience.

Mooli Lahad PhD PhD
Professor of Psychology and Dramatherapy
Head of the MA program in Dramatherapy, Tel Hai College, Israel

Note
Professor Lahad's work in trauma prevention and recovery is developed in Section Three 'Identifying Coping Strengths in Children & Young People who have Experienced Trauma'.

Section One

Introduction

How can we understand traumas and the impact they may have on people? How can we grasp 'Post-Traumatic-Stress-Disorder' (PTSD) and its capacity to stop children, teenagers and adults from being able to live happy and contented lives? The impact of trauma can affect individuals at every level, and as in the example of Janice (Case Study 1, p.8), it can distort the whole of our lives unless there is appropriate intervention. There are many ways of addressing trauma, as this book illustrates, but just sometimes, a teacher who is willing to listen or a care worker who has time for telling a child a story can make all the difference. Above all we are supporting children and teenagers to discover hope, and with hope they will be able to trust themselves and the people around them.

It is easy to say that 'time will heal' or 'pull yourself together' or 'it's all over now', as if the trauma and associated PTSD can be shaken off and forgotten about. Much was written about trauma in the period after the Two World Wars. Indeed soldiers were shot for showing 'cowardice' in the face of war, when it was later realised that they had PTSD and could not function at any level. We need to remember that there are three immediate responses to extreme shock and fear. They are the three Fs:

FREEZE: the person is frozen to the spot and unable to function or respond to instructions. They are literally rooted to the place where they stand, and threats or violence make no difference.

FLIGHT: the person's sole response is escape and they will find every possible way to remove themselves from the traumatic environment. If someone is locked up or restrained when they try to run away it will make their condition worse.

FIGHT: the person tries to fight back, even if it impossible to win. A child will hurl themselves at an adult who is abusing them or an adult will take on a gang of bullies.

The person may then continue these responses, even when there is no trauma, but a possible trigger such as a sound, smell or image. We only have to remember how powerful memories can be triggered by smell: fresh ground coffee, cinnamon, roses, bergamot can all take us back to a pleasant experience where we smelt these things before. Therefore it is understandable if a smell or other sensory experience can take us back to the traumatic event and trigger the coping response. For example a child who had been beaten and had a plaster stuck over her mouth would shake with fear if she could smell the particular antiseptic that is impregnated in such plasters; a teenager who escaped from a burning car would run away in terror if he smelt burning petrol or oil, a scent that is very common in garage workshops. Furthermore, it was a long time before he could get into a car or any other small space.

The origins of the word trauma seem to be from the same word in Greek, meaning: a physical or psychic wound, appearing in writings as early as 1693, according to Chambers Etymological Dictionary (2003). It has now come to mean the long-lasting effect of a major shock to an individual or to a group of people.

The trauma may be physical shock following a serious accident or psychological shock, for example, after a tsunami, or an incident of personal abuse or major loss. Whole communities can be traumatised by a disaster, or the ripples of impact can reach far beyond an individual's experience. In general terms the impact of trauma can affect individuals of any age (even pre-birth) from babies to elderly people, families, small communities, whole countries. The trauma of the Holocaust has affected Jewish people, Roma populations and other minorities for several generations.

Children can be traumatised through continuous beatings or sexual abuse, or through neglect and lack of nurture. This may seem a very large grouping of potentially trauma-inducing incidents, and I think they can be usefully re-grouped into the following seven categories:

1 Caused by nature: tsunamis, floods, hurricanes, volcano eruptions
2 Caused by people: train, car and aircraft crashes, wars, terrorism and genocide
3 Inflicted by one or more people on others: rape, torture, intimidation, and kidnap
4 Inflicted specifically by 'carers' in institutions: physical and emotional neglect, ridicule, lack of nurture, bullying and cruelty
5 Inflicted by one person continuously on another: sexual abuse, beatings, emotional abuse, bullying and cruelty
6 Inflicted by parents, the people who are supposed to care and nurture: physical, emotional and sexual abuse, neglect
7 The impact of major and often unexpected loss of attachments: death of parents, grandparents or children; loss or death of best friends, pets, home; divorce or separation

It is teachers, carers and classroom support workers who may notice the early signs of trauma, especially in category 7, which could be described as the impact of life transitions that are not contained in the normal day-to-day management of loss and subsequent grieving. For example, how alert are we to the shock of moving from a small school to a large one, in a new area, where no friends have gone with us? However we all need to be vigilant for changes in behaviour, signs of bruising, lack of concentration, self-harming and day-dreaming that can result from trauma in all of the groups 4–7. Bullying may be happening within the school, and staff may observe that there are indicators of some form of trauma response. Children and young people who have experienced trauma from groups 1–3 are more likely to be understood by the larger society who are more used to dealing with such crises and atrocities.

It is important, however, to be clear that not all shocking experiences and tragedies cause trauma. Many children and teenagers have resilient families or personal strengths that help them cope with unexpected events. Michael Rutter (1997) in a longitudinal study found that 80 percent of children coped with traumatic events providing they had one coping parent. Children and young people who are able to report bullying or intimidation will rarely have lasting effects. This of course is providing that they are 'heard' by teacher or parent, and appropriate action is taken. Although schools are supposed by law to have an effective anti-bullying strategy in place, it is not always made use of. It is not helpful for bullied children to be told 'just ignore it' or 'hit back' or 'it will toughen you up' (Hickson 2011). This book is the best anti-bullying resource that I have discovered.

I personally remember only too well the feelings of dread of going to junior school and secondary school as I knew the bullying would continue. My parents employed the 'look the other way' or 'take no notice' type of response. And yes, I found my own 'classic' coping strategy through becoming the clown or by appeasement through gifts.

We can never make everything 'all right' for other people. We can hold and contain them, allow them time and space for healing, and indeed work with creative ideas to try and break the cycle of traumatic experience. However, we also need to be aware of our own traumas that may have happened to us at some time in our lives. It is very important that we hold on to our own experience and don't let it get in the way of our work with others. Their experience is different, and is not helped if we say things like, 'I had the same experience …' or 'What really worked for me was …' or 'Time to move on and forget all that …'

Children and teenagers who have been taken into care because of abuse or neglect, need to be able to recover from the abuse through appropriate activities or counselling. It is not enough to say, 'You can leave all that behind you'! A carer who is not conversant with the impact of lost attachments can seem oblivious to the sudden trauma that can make an impact on a child's emotional life. Furthermore, if abusive parents are made 'all bad' by carers or other professionals, what is the impact on the child, who is after all part of both of these parents? A child or teenager needs to understand that they have inherited something positive from their parents even if they did wicked things.

We need to be alert when we see someone who is not coping: the baby who sleeps all the time, the 'good' and compliant child, the switched off or disaffected teenager, the silent adult, or the weeping frail adult. How can we make a difference, in order to achieve something of the contentment that is everyone's birthright?

Introduction

Who Should Run These Sessions?

When there has been a major disaster such as a train crash or shooting or flood, there are usually trained professionals who are skilled in providing appropriate support and counselling. However, there have been times when communities have resented so much external interference (for example after the Lockerbie bombing). Yet after the Aberfan tragedy there were pleas for help to cope with so much trauma and loss.

Many therapists and counsellors are also trained to work with the effects of trauma. However they are not always available, without delay, to work with children and teenagers in homes and schools. Teachers and care workers with brief training and appropriate support, are able to work with individuals and groups through the various techniques in this book. There are basic principles to follow which are described below, and everyone must be alert, as stated below, to possible disclosures that need further action. All schools and homes have a protocol for dealing with disclosure of abuse.

Planning the Sessions

Frequency: If possible there should be a minimum of three sessions, with time for homework in between. Once a week for three weeks is ideal, although it maybe necessary to plan for 5 or 6 weeks if the trauma is severe.

Length of Time: Usually one and a half hours for a group is sufficient for focussed work and concentration. An individual session would last for 45-50 minutes.

Individual or Group? Generally I recommend groupwork because participants are supported by each other and are reassured they are not the only one to have experienced the trauma

Similar Experiences or Different?

Although some groups may be planned for members who have been through the same experience, (school bus crash or unexpected fire for example), it can prove helpful to bring together people who have experienced different types of trauma. It widens everyone's understanding and encourages support and insight. It is also useful to think of running a group where perhaps only a small number of participants have experienced immediate traumas, but other members may have had similar experienced in the past. Some may not have experienced trauma but would be ideal individuals to learn how to be supportive and understanding to those who are having difficulties.

Introduction

Choice of Techniques

Cautions

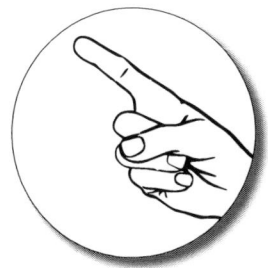

As teachers and facilitators it is important to be as vigilant as we can about possible disclosures. In trauma work it can happen that the nurture and care can trigger new responses and disclosures about abuse or neglect. Practitioners need to be aware of the policy of their school or organisation for handling disclosures, and to be knowledgeable about the school's anti-bullying policy. Furthermore it may be that one trauma can hide another one, as described in the example of Janice and her 'out-of-body-experience' (see p.8).

Therapists are required to have regular supervision of their practice, no matter how much experience they have, and this provides support for them, and protection for clients. If supervision is not available, meeting with colleagues perhaps once a month, or every six weeks, can help trauma workers feel less isolated in their very demanding work.

Health and Safety issues need to address the rules of the particular organisation. Environments need to be safe and the use of candles and incense (Section Six) need to be executed with care. Of course, it is inappropriate to use candles if a trauma has been caused by a fire.

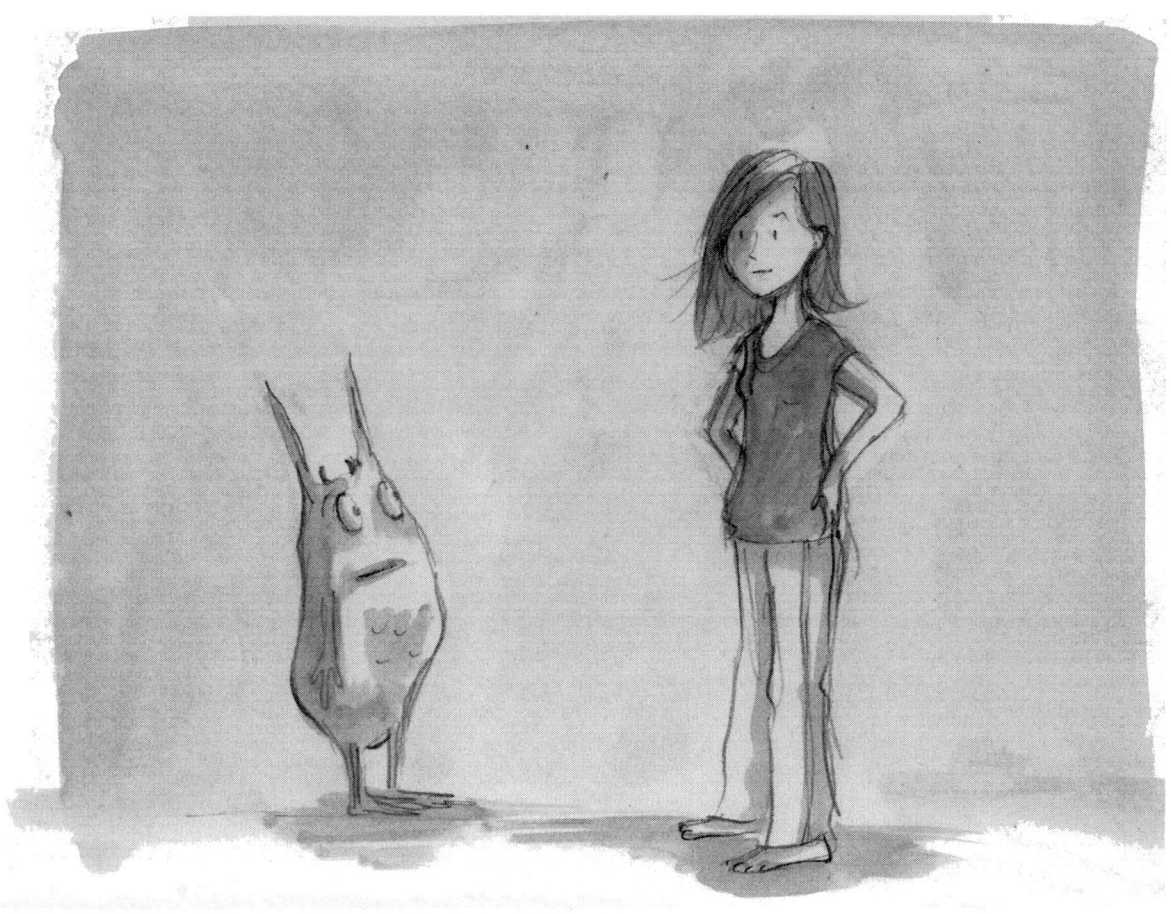

Welcoming the Monster

Section Two

The Building Blocks of Recovery: the Body & the Brain

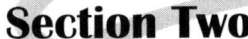

Responses to trauma as described above can be either: 'freeze', 'flight' or 'fight': either the person is frozen to the spot and unable to move, runs away or fights back. These three responses to a traumatic incident or experience are activated in the brain by the amygdala, which is part of the limbic system and situated in the midbrain. The amygdala immediately communicates to us what is dangerous or to be avoided. It is the part of the brain that is needed for survival and it reminds us to eat and sleep and seek shelter, as well as alerting us to potential danger. As Sunderland (2006) describes:

> *There are several genetically ingrained emotional systems deep in the lower brain, and knowledge of these systems is a key to good parenting. The systems are RAGE, FEAR, SEPARATION DISTRESS, SEEKING CARE, PLAY (and LUST which is not developed in children). (p.24)*

She goes on to say, and I think her words are important for everyone concerned with children and young people, not only parents:

> *The Rage, Fear and Separation Systems are already set up at birth to support a baby's survival. They are designed to be so in order to save infants from being eaten by predators, and to keep them close to a parent. The potential dangers in a modern world are very different but nevertheless can easily trigger one or more of these systems in your baby's brain. (p.24)*

It is understandable, therefore when the fear and separation emotional systems are triggered if a mother walks out of the room, as a small infant does not yet have a higher, rational brain to understand what is going on.

Similarly the lower brain also houses the traumatic memories associated with traumatic and fearful past events and may alert us, even when the event is past. Many individuals have recurring freeze, flight, fight responses, despite the passage of time, and this is known as PTSD (Post-Traumatic Stress Disorder). As well as sensory stimulus, people may also be reminded by an intrusive memory or nightmare of the traumatic event, and their stress symptoms are reactivated. These can include sweating, difficulties in sleeping, increased heart beats (palpitations), tearfulness, irritability, feelings of shame and worthlessness, overwhelming guilt, extreme fear, depression, lack of concentration or motivation, obsessive routines, and dissociation.

> ## Case Study 1
> This is an example of an adult with long-term PTSD which illustrates how childhood trauma can affect someone for life, unless there is recognition of the trauma and appropriate treatment put in place. In this situation, the traumatic events had taken place both at birth and during childhood, but the former did not emerge until several months in to therapy.
>
> 'Janice', aged 55, consulted about her dissociation or 'out of body experiences', that would overwhelm her in many public as well as home situations. She felt completely incapable of controlling her bodily reactions of tension, stomach cramps and permanent frowns. She was unable to find the stressor that would provoke her to go out of her own body. She was frightened of sleeping because she would wake up in terror and out of control, and it affected her work and social life as she was scared of unprovoked episodes. She attempted to impose total control over her body through diet, exercise, and cleanliness.
>
> She told me that I probably would not want to know about the beatings as no other therapist had thought them important. She had been systematically beaten with a leather whip by her father, who had brutalised the whole family in drunken rages. There were many triggers for her dissociation; for example as a child, the family would sit waiting at the meal table for the father to return. They would know he was arriving when they heard the scrunch on gravel of his car, all the children would sit up straight and fresh hot food was put on the table. The father would come in and often turn the dining table over or take the food and throw it against the wall, while shouting abuse, but sometimes would just join the family for the evening meal. The scrunch of wheels or feet on gravel still caused her anxiety and could cause an out-of-body episode.

Out-of-body experience is common when a person has been unable to escape a brutal or sexual assault; it is a freeze response that can later be triggered by any associated stimulus. When one cannot escape from the trauma, the brain's coping mechanism enables one to 'escape' from the body that is being assaulted, at least in consciousness.

In Janice's situation, falling asleep meant that she had lost control, and the proximity of people in public meant the possibility of stranger-danger. Basically she needed to be vigilant at all times and in all places. However when she was able to mother herself and create her own 'safe-place', she was able to develop greater 'trust of the other'. Although we initially worked with her feelings about the beatings and the generalised fear in the family at unprovoked violent episodes, an early trauma was then remembered in a quite unexpected way.

She brought in a newspaper article about a terrorist attack where a pregnant woman had been murdered. This reminded her of the stories surrounding her own birth, where the midwife, herself pregnant, had been murdered on her way to deliver Janice. It slowly emerged that she had literally been born in to a 'circle of fear', as there were armed and ruthless terrorists surrounding the area where her family lived. She was often hidden in a cupboard in case there was a raid on the house. In Janice's situation there seemed no basis for a trusting attachment with either of her parents, as her father beat her and her mother did not protect her, but also the fear of attack rendered the whole family helpless, so she was unable even to trust her environment. Trust seemed a key theme for Janice in all of her work, even to testing me as her therapist, as she came to see me and then stopped and then came again.

The work of Erikson (1951/1995) shows the importance of the development of trust during the first eighteen months of life. He maintains that the first developmental stage of the child is that of acquiring trust or mistrust. Trust comes about through a healthy attachment relationship which is discussed below.

In my therapeutic practice, I integrate a combination of body work (self-soothing, massage, sensory play, movement and relaxation); telling of personal stories through objects in the sand-tray; dramatic play where metaphoric and symbolic scenes are represented through movement 'body-sculpts' and role play or drama. Time and again for Janice there would be images of total chaos and destruction, like a black hole where she would be swallowed up in the chaos and destruction, or destroyed by the power of the invaders. Much of the time there were accompanying feelings of shame, guilt and blame.

What was helpful was her developing capacity to reflect in a mindful way on her own journey through the day and night, which slowly imparted a feeling of her own control; the following methods assisted her to move forward:

a Learning to self-soothe, and to care for herself in a nurturing way;
b Expressing her here-and-now feelings in the therapeutic sand tray with small toys and objects;
c Placing significant people on an empty chair and telling them what she had bottled up for so many years;
d Building larger than life 'sculpts' of the destructive elements in her life;
e Recognising her own journey in a variety of stories, and especially in 'The Hero's Journey' (p.124), and 'The Transformation of Sedna' (see p.133);
f Finding ways to go beyond her body in creative ways such as joining a singing group and a dance class.

It was important for both of us to learn the significance of the theme of trust and also of control. There is more about the 'Myth of Sedna', and Janice and other trauma group members in Section Nine 'Healing Stories'.

Attachment

Attachment is the primary bond between mother and child that is usually established during the first two years of life. The most important pioneer of attachment theory and innovation was John Bowlby (1988), who together with Mary Ainsworth established the basis of the future understanding of attachment. Initially Bowlby's work was scorned by the then current psychoanalytic closed circle, and he was ousted from the inner membership of Freud's disciples for his heresy. Bowlby showed extreme courage in the face of such hostility. Prevailing attitudes at the time wished to give credence to the idea that children and adults had fantasies about their abuse, rather than it existing in reality. Nannies and early boarding school were considered appropriate for healthy child rearing. Bowlby himself learned from his own trauma at being suddenly separated from a beloved nanny and being placed in a boarding school at a young age. This early damaging experience became the basis on which he built his theory of attachment.

The development of secure attachments is particularly important during the first two years of life (Jennings 2011), and my own observations suggest that it also begins to be established during pregnancy. Awareness of the unborn child from conception onwards means that a relationship is beginning to form even prior to birth. The awareness of the unborn child and simple playful interactions such as stroking, patting, singing and storytelling contribute to a creative and playful attachment relationship.

Recent research in neuroscience (Gerhardt 2004) has shown that 'good enough' attachment makes an important impact on the brain, and the quality of the primary attachment relationship will influence all future relationships, both personal and social. Whereas early psychological opinion was divided between whether nature or nurture was the most important factor in a child's development. The geneticists believed that biological inheritance, what we are born with, played the most significant role; whereas those who believed in care and nurture, thought how a baby was looked after was more significant.

Gerhardt (2004) says that:

> *Babies are like the raw material for a self. Each one comes with a genetic blueprint and a unique range of possibilities. There is a body programmed to develop in certain ways, but by no means on an automatic programme. The baby is an interactive project not a self-powered one. The baby human organism has various systems ready to go, but many more that are incomplete and will only develop through another human input.* (p.18)

Attachment is an 'interactive project' and consists of the social playfulness between mother and new-born child from birth. If a primary attachment is not possible with the mother, then other significant adults can take on that role: dad, grandma, auntie and so on. The importance of consistency during the first twelve months or so of life cannot be over-emphasised.

There are continuing discoveries in neuroscience that inform us about the influence of the brain on childhood attachment, and the importance of nurture (Gerhardt 2004). There is intense debate about mirror neurons (Whitehead 2001) which fire when certain actions are observed by infants, and are thought to contribute to group activities such as dance and ritual and 'setting a good example' (Jennings 2011). However, there is still continued debate on what can be generalised from neuroscience in education and therapy. These discoveries influence how children grow up to behave, and that attachment has a profound effect on the growth of the brain and the security of the child (Sunderland 2006). Again this is directed at parents but has overall relevance to this topic:

> *Everything your baby experiences with you as his parent will forge connections between the cells in his higher brain. The human brain is specifically designed this way so that it can be wired up to adapt to a particular environments in which it finds itself. This adaptability works for or against the well-being of the child. If, for example, a child has a bullying parent, he can start to adapt to living in a bullying world, with all manner of changes in brain structure and brain chemical systems, which may result in hyper-vigilance, heightened aggression or fear reactions, or heightened attack/ defence impulses in the reptilian part of his brain.* (p.22)

It is also important to be aware of the loss of attachments in later life. Elderly people may have lost their spouse, their homes, their pets and any one of these losses can be traumatic. People who are developing dementia are aware of their failing faculties, and family members are mourning the loss of the person they used to know (Creative Care 2012). Losses that are not coped with as part of the usual life-cycle of 'birth, growing up, education, working life, parenthood, grandparenthood, death' can be traumatic for individuals, families and communities.

In trauma work, understanding the importance of attachment is central for guiding methods of intervention. In major disasters, many people will have lost significant attachment figures, sometimes their entire family. The loss of parents and spouses, especially in unexpected circumstances, often prompts a trauma response. Children who have had inappropriate attachment experiences with a parent or parents, including abuse of all kinds, will experience trauma, which is often pervasive. Similarly the child who has been neglected and rejected will usually need trauma intervention in order to experience an appropriate attachment, including nurture and sensory play.

Early Developmental Attachment and Play Sequencing

Neuro-Dramatic-Play

Neuro-Dramatic-Play (NDP) forms the basis of playful attachment between mother and unborn child and mother and new-born child. The important time-frame is from six months before birth until six months after birth. NDP is unique in focussing on the playful nature of pregnancy, and links it to the dramatised and playful attachment after the birth (Jennings 2011).

Through play and drama, NDP emphasises a combination of basic trust (Erikson 1995), security and ritual, together with sensory stimulation, physical movement, exploration and risk (Jennings 2011; 2012). Ritual and risk form the basis of children feeling safe in the world, as well as a desire to explore the world. Although the infant experiences ritualistic behaviour before birth, with the patterns of the mother's routine, experiences of light and dark, changes in temperature, it is the birth itself that is the first major ritual in a child's life. Ancient societies had their own fertility goddesses and ritual practice which made childbirth very different from today's experience. However, with an increase in the use of birthing pools and home births, there is some increase in awareness of the ritual of birth, and the importance of transitions.

Neuro-Dramatic-Play consists of sensory play, rhythmic play and dramatic play, which all take place during the crucial six month periods (Jennings 2011; 2012). This early attachment period has a profound effect on the child's later development.

Neuro-Dramatic-Play enables children to become more independent and self-reliant. It affirms their identity and self-esteem, and the building of social relationships. It helps to form the basis of their later resilience and coping skills.

Neuro-Dramatic-Play can be used as an important intervention for working with children and young people who have been traumatised through disaster, accident, loss or abuse. Indeed NDP principles can be applied at any age from the very young to the very old.

When people are traumatised the physical and psychological impact can take different forms. For example, a child may appear to be coping but is having recurrent nightmares or has lost their rhythm of life (everything is completed at a much slower pace, or very fast as if there is no time to be lost). Some individuals may seem cut off from their emotions or their feelings spill out everywhere and with everybody. The use of sensory, rhythmic and dramatic playfulness of NDP assists a child or group of children to reconnect with their capacity for healing play. There are NDP techniques and exercises for trauma in the practical Sections Three to Nine.

Early Developmental Patterning and Attachment

Embodiment-Projection-Role

The three stages of EPR are:

- Embodiment: birth to 12 months (everything is experienced through the body)
- Projection: 13 months to 3 years (toys and media beyond the body are explored)
- Role: 3 years to 7 years (roles and stories are developed in dramatic play).

These age-stages are not absolute as they occur at different times in different children, but all stages need to be completed for confident maturation and emotional resilience. Embodiment–Projection–Role is a developmental sequencing that I have been expanding and exploring since the mid-1980s. The above three stages seem to occur across cultures in more or less the same framework. Initially infants are focused completely on their bodies and the body of their mothers: food and nurture, sensory play, singing games and so on move through the first twelve months as gradually there is an interest in the world beyond the body. This leads into the projection stage where objects and events beyond the body arouse intense interest. Play with toys and puzzles grows and more complete interactions emerge such as imitation of scenes with a doll's house or puppets. This indicates, usually around 3–4 years that there is another move towards the role stage with an increase in playing-out stories and events. EPR is extremely useful for structuring lessons and workshops as it assists children and teenagers who may have missed out on the stages to regain these crucial areas of development.

However, all the stages in NDP and EPR can be re-visited in education, therapeutic play and arts therapies for children who have been subject to trauma.

Neuro-Dramatic-Play overlaps with this second developmental paradigm: 'Embodiment-Projection-Role' (EPR), (Jennings 1990; 1998; 2004; 2011) that starts from birth. EPR incorporates and expands the sensory-rhythmic-dramatic developmental sequencing, and shows how a child is involved in a series of dramatic scenarios and activities between birth and the age of 7 years. NDP develops from 6 months before birth to six months after birth, so NDP and EPR overlap by about 6 months. The timing of this overlap is crucial as it encompasses the 'dramatic response', otherwise known as the 'as if' response of the small infant, when trying to imitate the expression on the mother's face. This usually happens within a few hours of birth. Most play by small infants is dramatic play, with changes in expression, vocal sounds and a persistence for imitation. Both NDP and EPR show that dramatic play and the 'as if' are central to human development.

Case Study 2

Trauma and Macbeth

Reflections on a fictive case-history

On seeing recently Shakespeare's play of 'Macbeth', I was struck by how many of the situations and responses mirrored everything we are discussing in relation to trauma. It would be helpful to watch a DVD of the play just to heighten your own awareness of trauma and response, remembering that it was written and understood long before trauma work became a profession. No wonder people refer to 'Dr Theatre' or the theatre being a place of healing, as well as entertainment!

Having been rewarded for a successful battle by the King, Macbeth meets three witches who predict his future, confirming that finally he will become King. Macbeth believes the witches and now makes sure that he removes anyone who might stand in his way. However, the main activist is Lady Macbeth, who goads him into continuing the murders, and even commits one herself.

The following are examples of trauma responses from the script of Macbeth.

Flight

The scene when murderers attack Banquo and his son Fleance who are waylaid on their road home.

> *Enter Banquo and Fleance with a torch*
> **2 Murderer:** A light, a light!
> **3 Murderer:** 'Tis he.
> **1 Murderer:** Stand to't
> **Banquo:** It will rain tonight
> **1 Murderer:** Let it come down.
> (*First Murderer strikes out light, while the others assault Banquo*)
> **Banquo:** O, treachery! Fly, good Fleance, fly, fly, fly!
>
> Act III, scene iii, 13–17

Fight

The scene of the slaughter of Macduff's children in typically illustrates a fight response. Macbeth sends murderers to kill the wife of Macduff and their two children. The young boy challenges the murderer and is promptly stabbed.

> *Enter Murderers*
> **Mur:** Where is your husband?
> **Lady Mac:** I hope, in no place so unsanctified,
> Where such as thou mays't find him.
> **Mur:** He's a traitor
> **Son:** Thou liest, thou shag-hair'd villain!
> **Mur:** What you egg? (*Stabbing him*)
> Young fry of treachery!
> **Son:** He has kill'd me mother;
> Run away, I pray you! (*He dies*)
>
> Act IV, scene xi, 79–87

Freeze

Towards the end of the play a servant comes to Macbeth with a message which he is scared to deliver, made more dramatic by the previous speech where Macbeth says he will never doubt or fear!

> *Enter a Servant, who is obviously pale with fear and stuttering …*
> **Macbeth:** The devil damn thee black, thou cream-fac'd loon!
> Where gott'st thou that goose look?
> **Servant:** There is ten thousand …
> **Macbeth:** Geese, villain?
> **Servant:** Soldiers, Sir
> *Macbeth is so angry with him, calling him linen cheeked and whey faced and eventually dismissing him.*
>
> Act V, scene iii, 11–15

There are not only these examples of fight, flight and freeze responses but the following also show typical responses to trauma.

After the murder of Banquo, the Macbeths hold a banquet for the nobles, and Macbeth has a hallucination of seeing Banquo sitting in his chair, shaking his bloodied hair, 'Never shake thy gory locks at me'; every time he mentions Banquo's name the 'ghost' re-appears and Macbeth gets more and more terrified, finally saying 'hence, horrible shadow'.

However, probably the most dramatic image is Lady Macbeth's sleep-walking scene, following her murder of two of the King's guards, and Macbeth's murder of King Duncan. She is deeply asleep while she is walking, is very agitated and rubbing her hands, 'Out, damned spot! Out I say' she says, and then 'Yet who would have thought the old man to have so much blood in him?', and later, 'What's done cannot be undone'.

Act V scene i

The doctor who has observed her sleep-walking says: 'More needs she the divine than the physician'. There is a theme of sleep running through the play and Macbeth says he heard a voice cry out: 'Sleep no more! Macbeth does murder Sleep – the innocent sleep that knits up the ravell'd sleeve of care.

Act II scene ii

These are just a few of the scenes and situations that illustrate some of the major symptoms and responses to trauma in Macbeth, and most importantly show how sleep disturbance is a major factor in PTSD. This will be dealt with in more detail in Section 6 'Night-fears & Nightmares'.

Section Three

Identifying Coping Strengths in Children & Young People who have Experienced Trauma

Activities & Worksheets

Activities

3.1 A 'BASIC Ph' Assessment of Coping Strategies in Young People, Part 1
3.2 A 'BASIC Ph' Assessment, Part 2
3.3 Who Else is in My Picture?
3.4 My Personal Skills & Strengths
3.5 Remembering to be Playful
3.6 Story Circle or Mandala
3.7 Circles of Protection (1)
3.8 Circles of Protection (2)
3.9 Chains of Qualities & Strengths

Worksheets

3a Story in Six Parts
3b Story Circle or Mandala
3c Circles of Protection: Personal
3d Circles of Protection: Social
3e Chains of Qualities & Strengths

Section Three

Identifying Coping Strengths in Children & Young People who have Experienced Trauma: Using the Six-Part Story Approach

How to understand people's coping strengths through the Six-Part Story Method

Mooli Lahad devised a method he has termed 'BASIC Ph' for assessing coping and resilience skills in children and teenagers who have suffered trauma and loss. It grew out of his observations of children in Israel who were in bomb shelters during rocket attacks, and their different ways of coping with stress. His assessment is based on what a child can do, rather than what they cannot do. He noticed that children had very individual ways of dealing with stressful situations, and he began to classify their different responses. Initially these were not organised activities but things children chose to do in order to cope with the here and now. He describes the six major ways of coping that all people will activate in a crisis or traumatic situation. This is Positive Psychology and Mindfulness working at their best. The following outline of the method gives basic instructions for its use and it is developed further in Lahad 2000, Jennings 2004 and Lahad et al 2013.

As described in the Introduction, there are several ways to cope with stress and trauma. Lahad et al (2013) demonstrate that most individuals have their own particular way of coping, and it is possible to assess someone's coping strength. Lahad suggests that there are six different ways of coping, the ways in which we 'meet the world', he termed these the BASIC Ph methods of coping.

To summarise, Lahad states that people will deal with their trauma through one or more of the following, though they are likely to have a dominant coping mode.

a Cognition and thinking routines (usually requiring lots of factual information);
b Emotional and affective responses (often needing nurture and comfort)

Introduction

c Social and group activities (other people join in games or social activities)

d Imagination and daydreaming (using art activities, poetry, stories and drama)

e Belief system of a particular religion, or self-esteem or a belief in the order of life;

f Physical activities such as sports, games, dance routines.

For instance, a child might well have (c) and (f) as strengths – sports are mainly social activities, so this would combine the physical with the social.

There are six modes and if the letters are re-arranged in order of Belief, Affect, Social, Imagination, Cognition and Physical, the first letters give us BASIC Ph, which is the name Lahad has given to the techniques and their underpinning theory.

BASIC Ph can be used for assessing someone's coping strengths, usually before interventions take place. For some children it may be that they need to have settled into some creative or relaxing activities before beginning the assessment. It is important that this does not seem like a formal task that is making yet further demands on an individual. It can be incorporated as a part of general art work or story work.

It is also helpful for professionals themselves to try out the BASIC Ph exercise and discover their own coping strengths. Remember it is the strength that is the main coping strength in the story that is important.

Activities

3.1 A 'BASIC Ph' Assessment of Coping Strategies in Young People Part 1

This assessment of a young person's coping strategies is designed to be carried out over two sessions to allow time for discussion and feedback.

Suitable for both Children and Teenagers

Resources: Plain paper, coloured pens and pencils, writing pens, folder for keeping course work, and notebook for writing and drawing, fleece, Worksheet 3a 'Story in Six Parts' (optional).

Ambience: Calm and comfortable room, drinking water available, lack of external noise or interruption.

Explanation: Whether working with an individual or a small group, introduce the idea of storytelling and how it is possible to tell stories through several pictures and/or words, drawn or written in a series of boxes.

The story is about a main character (1), and whether he or she can achieve the important task (2) they have set themselves. There is something or someone trying to stop the character achieving their task (3). Is there anyone who can assist them (4)? So what happens next (5)? How does the story end (6)?

It is important to reassure the children or teenagers that they do not have to be good at drawing in order to show the important elements of the story.

Task: First the children or teenagers can either use Worksheet 3a or divide their piece of paper into six sections of equal size (it is important to emphasise the boxes should be of equal size or they will may be too big or small and it will be difficult to fit them in); they may choose to fold the paper into six, or draw six boxes. Then work through the six stages of the story, one at a time, encouraging the young person to draw or write their idea of what happens in each box. They can take as much time as necessary, and ask any questions they wish as they go along. It is important that you repeat the instructions rather than prompting as a response to questions. Remember that this is a story for assessing coping skills, not for therapeutic work.

Invite the child or teenager to tell you the story in their own words, using their pictures as an illustration of what they are telling you. You will need to listen in several ways:

- What tone of voice does the child use?
- What is the context in which the child tells the story?
- How near or far from the story does the child seem to be?
- Is it a reworking of a well-known story in their own words, or does it have significant variations that you need to pay attention to?
- Is it a completely new story that has come out of the child's imagination?

Write the story down as the child tells it to you, and then read it back to them to make sure they are happy that you have got it right.

Explain that everyone should think about their story and what they think their strengths are before the next session. Share stories with a partner or in the whole groups if there are fewer than five people.

Ending: encourage relaxation with the fleece and breathing exercises (see Section 4).

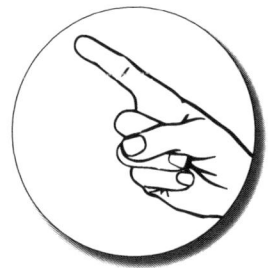

Preparation before next time:

Make notes from what the children or teenagers have said and shown in their pictures from the following:

- *Belief: Are there expressions of a belief system in the story?*
- *Affect: What feelings are expressed, if any?*
- *Social: Are there other people in the story?*
- *Imagination: Has the story an imaginative context?*
- *Cognition: Does the story contain thoughts or concrete facts?*
- *Physical: Does the story include a physical solution or activity?*

By reading through the story you can see in which areas the child has strengths; for example, there may be little feeling, but a lot of thought and belief. It is important to note how the issue is solved (if at all). Looking at the pictures, think about what story is being created. What do you think the child's main coping strength is? It will be indicated by the strength that is actually used to solve the difficulty in the story they have created.

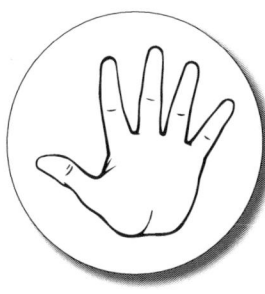

It is important that you do not approach this assessment in critical way. For example, if little emotion is shown in the story, it does not mean that the child or teenager is devoid of feelings; it shows they do not use their feelings as a coping strategy.

The table below can be used for recording your analysis of the story. It can be helpful to try it out on yourself and a couple of friends in order to feel comfortable with using it. Use Worksheet 3a to write your own Six Part Story and then consider the themes.

	Low	Medium	High
Belief			
Affect			
Social			
Imagination			
Cognition			
Physical			

Activity 3.1

3.2 'BASIC Ph' Assessment Part 2

Suitable for both Children and Teenagers

Resources: Worksheets or drawings from previous session, plain paper, coloured pens and pencils, writing pens, folder for course work and notebook for writing and drawing.

Ambience: Calm and comfortable room, drinking water available, lack of external noise or interruption.

Explanation: It is important to be able to share with the child or teenager their strengths and positively reinforce them. It is also important to accept their story even though it might not fit the formula. If there is a lot of violence in the story then it is possible to discuss that so much energy was used to deal with the difficulties. The idea of changing negative to positive energy can be introduced at a later session.

Task: Encourage group members to share any thoughts from the previous session about their drawings. What do they see as positive? Would they add anything to the story? Feedback their strengths and use a success approach of emphasising how well everyone has done in writing a story! For many it might be for the first time they have created a story, and it is important to give positive feedback for their creative efforts. Suggest they keep their art work and worksheets in their folders, and use their notebook as a diary to write or draw anything they wish about the work they are doing.

Ending: Suggest that everyone can decorate their folders in whatever way they would like, and write in their notebooks; allow time for relaxation with fleece and soothing music if appropriate, or a healing story (see Section Nine).

3.3 Who Else is in My Picture?

Suitable for both Children and Teenagers

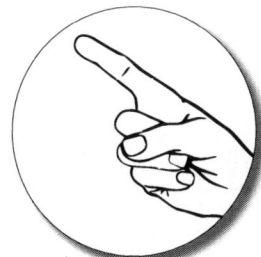

It is important for children and teenagers to experience how their traumatic experience is contained in the wider picture of their lives, and it can be especially helpful to think of a hero or heroine, this could be a real person or an imaginary person from a story or television programme.

Resources: Worksheets or drawings from previous session, plain paper, coloured pens and pencils, writing pens, folder for course work and notebook for writing and drawing, fleeces.

Ambience: Calm and comfortable room, drinking water available, lack of external noise or interruption.

Explanation: Discuss with the individual or group that there are various issues to be considered as well as the trauma itself. For example, does anyone have a hero or heroine who they really admire? What do they admire about that person? It could be the person who rescued them in a particular situation, or the person who cared for them in hospital.

Task: Invite everyone to draw a picture of their hero/heroine in their notebooks, making them as large as possible on the page. Think about the important qualities that the heroes have, and how they could be important in re-building lives; take time to colour the person and make them uniquely your own. Draw a speech bubble of helpful words that the person could be saying.

Ending: Share and discuss in the group the helpful words of the hero/heroine; and allow time for relaxation with fleece and soothing music if appropriate, or a healing story (see Section Nine).

3.4 My Personal Skills & Strengths

Suitable for both Children and Teenagers

Resources: plain paper, coloured pens and pencils, writing pens, folder for course work and notebook for writing and drawing, fleece and story book for closure.

Ambience: Calm and comfortable room, drinking water available, lack of external noise or interruption.

Explanation: It is important to reassure children and young people that they all have their own skills and strengths, something they are good at. Everyone has different skills, and sometimes when we are upset they can be forgotten.

Task: Invite everyone to think of skills that are very different, such as being a good listener, playing the guitar or being very observant of detail, you could write or draw a couple of examples on the board. Suggest that everyone draws cartoon or stick figures showing two of the skills they have in their notebooks.

Ending: Encourage group members to give feedback to each other about the skills they have; and allow time for relaxation with fleeces and soothing music if appropriate, or a healing story (see Section Nine).

3.5 Remembering to be Playful

Suitable for both Children and Teenagers

Resources: Plain paper, coloured pens and pencils, writing pens, folder for course work and notebook for writing and drawing, fleece and story book for closure.

Ambience: Calm and comfortable room, drinking water available, lack of external noise or interruption.

Explanation: Describe to the group how remembering to be playful is helpful when the world looks a bit grey or we are feeling miserable. It might be helpful to go for a run or play a sport or make something or paint a picture. There are lots of ways to be playful.

Task: Invite group member to come up with suggestions of different ways of being playful; some they have done in the past and some they have never tried. Encourage everyone to make a paper aeroplane and then send it across the room, on a count of 3 (most people are able to make an aeroplane and can help anyone who is struggling), and then send them back across the room.

Ending: Suggest everyone retrieves their own aeroplane (or makes another), and writes or draws on their plane one way of being playful; share in the group and put in folder; and allow time for relaxation with fleece and soothing music if appropriate, or a healing story (see Section Nine).

3.6 Story Circle or Mandala

Suitable for both Children and Teenagers

Resources: Plain paper, coloured pens and pencils, writing pens, folder for course work and notebook for writing and drawing, fleece and story book for closure, Worksheet 3b 'Story Circle or Mandala'.

Ambience: Calm and comfortable room, drinking water available, lack of external noise or interruption.

Explanation: Encourage discussion and feedback from the previous session and remind group members that they have thought about their different ways of coping, their hero/heroine, their skills and their playfulness (write the headings on the board as a reminder). Now they are going to put these different aspects of themselves into one picture. Give everyone a copy of the Worksheets. The Worksheet also includes a section about scary things and also what or who the young people believe in.

Task: Write and draw in the different sections. The group can use things they have created in previous sessions if they wish. For example in Box 1, they might put their hero/heroine for who or what they admire, and their paper aeroplane in 4, about playfulness.

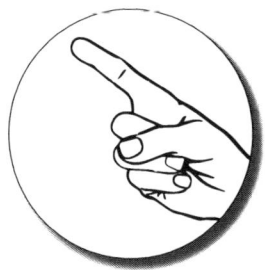

It is important that the participants are not set up to fail in this exercise. They may need more time to build up their confidence and playfulness through sensory work (Section Four), safety (Section Five) and games (included in Section Seven).

Ending: Encourage everyone to share one new positive thing they have learned about themselves during this exercise. What was the most difficult section to complete in the Mandala? Place pictures in folders and allow time for relaxation with fleece and soothing music if appropriate or a healing story (see Section Nine).

3.7 Circles of Protection (1)

Suitable for Teenagers

Resources: Plain paper, coloured pens and pencils, writing pens, folder for course work and notebook for writing and drawing, fleece and story book for closure, Worksheet 3c 'Circles of Protection: Personal'.

Ambience: Calm and comfortable room, drinking water available, lack of external noise or interruption.

Explanation: Everyone needs to feel safe and there are many ways we can help ourselves to feel comfort, (see Section Four Self-Soothing & Self-Care), as well as having comforting thoughts. Encourage group members to come up with different things that can be comforting and write them on the board, you could perhaps start the list e.g., with a soft bed and cover; a hot drink.

Task: Having shared comforting things, invite group members to draw, colour and write in Worksheet 3c. There are three circles and they can be filled in any order, with colours, words, pictures.

1. Inner circle, things that are comforting such as warm drinks, special foods, cuddly toys.
2. Middle circle, positive thoughts that give strengths and brighten up the worlds
3. Outer circle, people who are close family members, or friends who are supportive.

Ending: Invite everyone to share something from their middle circle (positive thoughts). Place pictures in folders and allow time for relaxation with fleeces and soothing music if appropriate or a healing story (see Section Nine).

3.8 Circles of Protection (2)

Suitable for both Children and Teenagers

Resources: Plain paper, coloured pens and pencils, writing pens, folder for course work and notebook for writing and drawing, fleece and story book for closure, Worksheet 3d 'Circles of Protection: Social'.

Ambience: Calm and comfortable room, drinking water available, lack of external noise or interruption.

Explanation: Everyone needs other people to support them and help them to feel safe; sometimes that may feel scary, and an imaginary friend can feel safer or perhaps a hero who you admire from film or television. What qualities do they have that you admire? Maybe people think of having those qualities themselves?

Task: Having supportive friends and family around us or imaginary friends can help us change our feelings: invite group members to colour and write in Worksheet 3d. There are three circles and they can be filled in any order, with colours, words and pictures:

1. Inner circle, imaginary friend or hero/heroine from sport, entertainment, music.
2. Best friend who is supportive and understanding.
3. Club or class of activities that involve concentration.

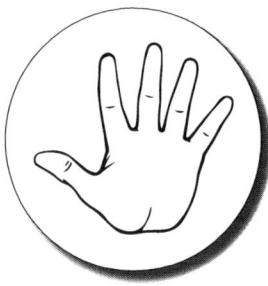

Some group members may feel that they do not have a best friend or that they are friendless. Try to intervene to stop this turning into a victim situation by saying for instance, 'Some people are still looking for a best friend – maybe someone who is in this group or at a sports club or in a class – so write or draw a best friend you would like to have'.

Ending: Share one important person in your picture with the whole group; place pictures in folder; and allow time for relaxation with fleece and soothing music if appropriate or a healing story (see Section Nine).

3.9 Chains of Qualities & Strengths

Suitable for Teenagers

Resources: Plain paper, coloured pens and pencils, writing pens, folder for course work and notebook for writing and drawing, fleece and notebook for closure, Worksheet 3e 'Chains of Qualities and Strengths'.

Ambience: Calm and comfortable room, drinking water available, lack of external noise or interruption.

Explanation: Describe, perhaps using colourful pictures of DNA, how our personal strengths, and the strengths and support we get from other people are intertwined in a shape rather like DNA helix. It is important to remind ourselves of our personal strengths as well as those we get from other people.

Task: Encourage everyone to colour Worksheet 3e, and follow through the two twisting chains of personal strengths and support we get from our friends. Experiment with using positive colours that weave in and out of each other.

Chain 1: Personal strengths, they may be ones discussed in previous exercises or individuals may feel they have acquired new ones.

Chain 2: Social strengths that we get from other people: maybe friends, maybe family.

Ending: Share one positive thing you have learnt in the group today, and write or draw it in notebooks; place pictures in folder; and allow time for relaxation with fleeces and soothing music if appropriate, or a healing story (see Section Nine).

Worksheet 3a

Story in Six Parts

Colour or write in each of the squares to create a story: 1 – main character, 2 – important task, 3 – block or sabotage, 4 – helper(s)?, 5 – what happens? 6 – How does the story end?

1	2
3	4
5	6

Worksheet 3b

Story Circle or Mandala

Colour and fill in the Mandala to tell your story, and decorate it in your favourite colours:

1. Who or what is your inspiration, or you admire?
2. What are you good at, or what were you good at?
3. What is scary or causes nightmares?
4. How can you be playful or creative?
5. Who or what do you believe in?

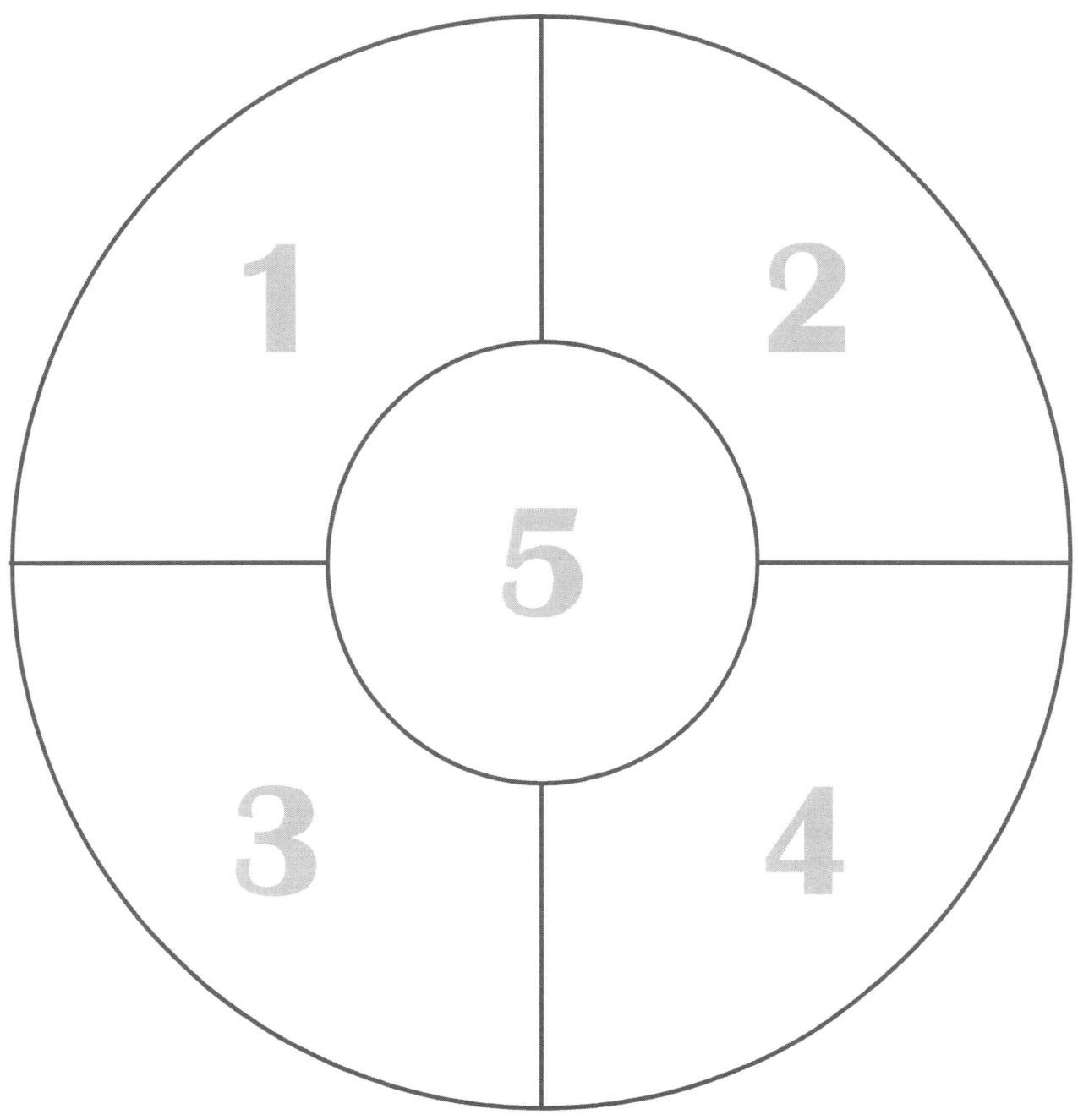

Worksheet 3c

Circles of Protection: Personal

Colour and write in the circles:

1. Things that are comforting or soothing such as warm drink, special food, cuddly toy
2. Positive thoughts that give strengths and brighten the world
3. People who are close in family or friends who are supportive.

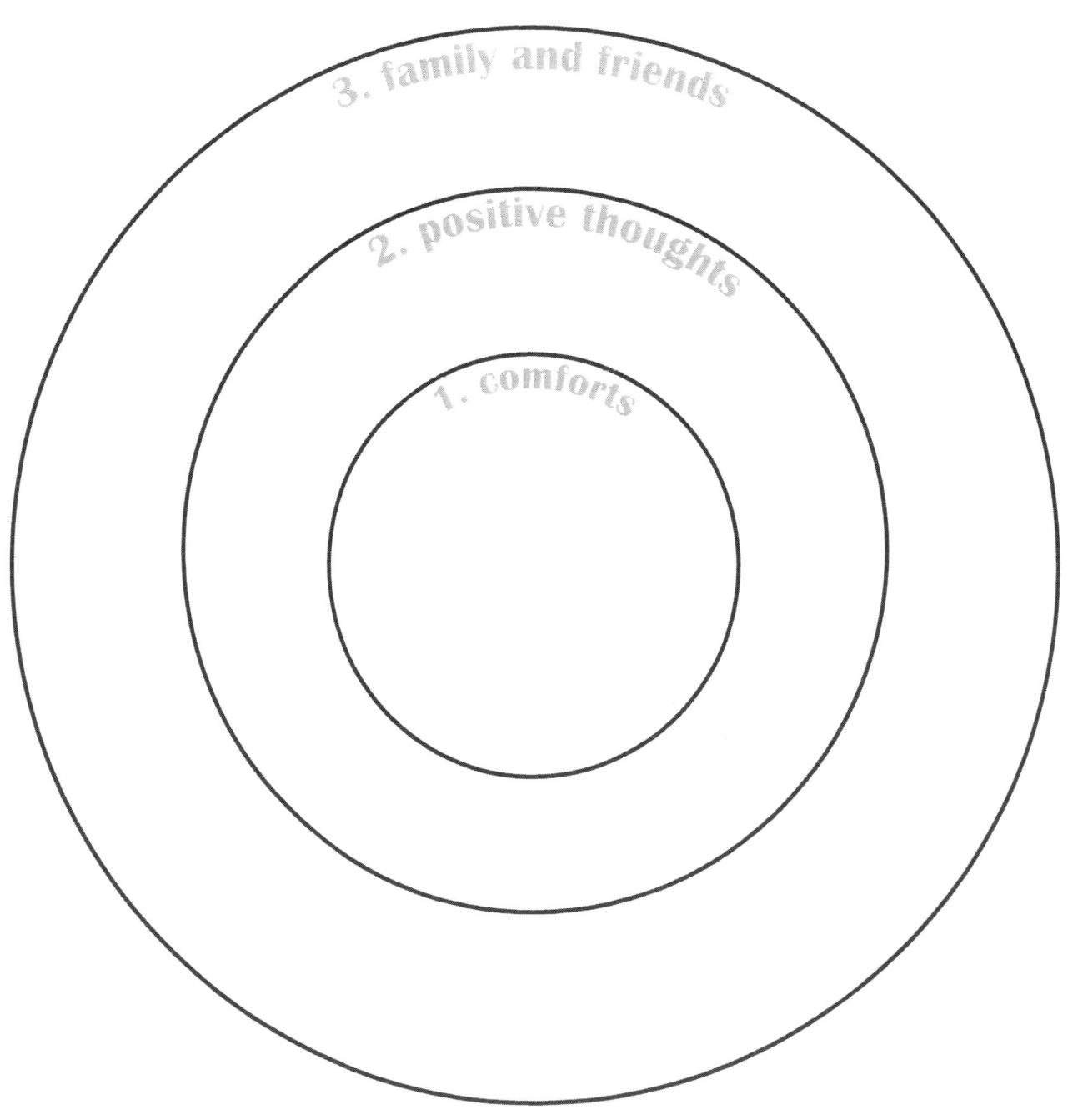

Worksheet 3d

Circles of Protection: Social

Colour and write in the circles:

1. Imaginary friend or a hero/heroine in sport, entertainment, music
2. Best friend who is supportive and understanding
3. Club or class of activities that involve concentration

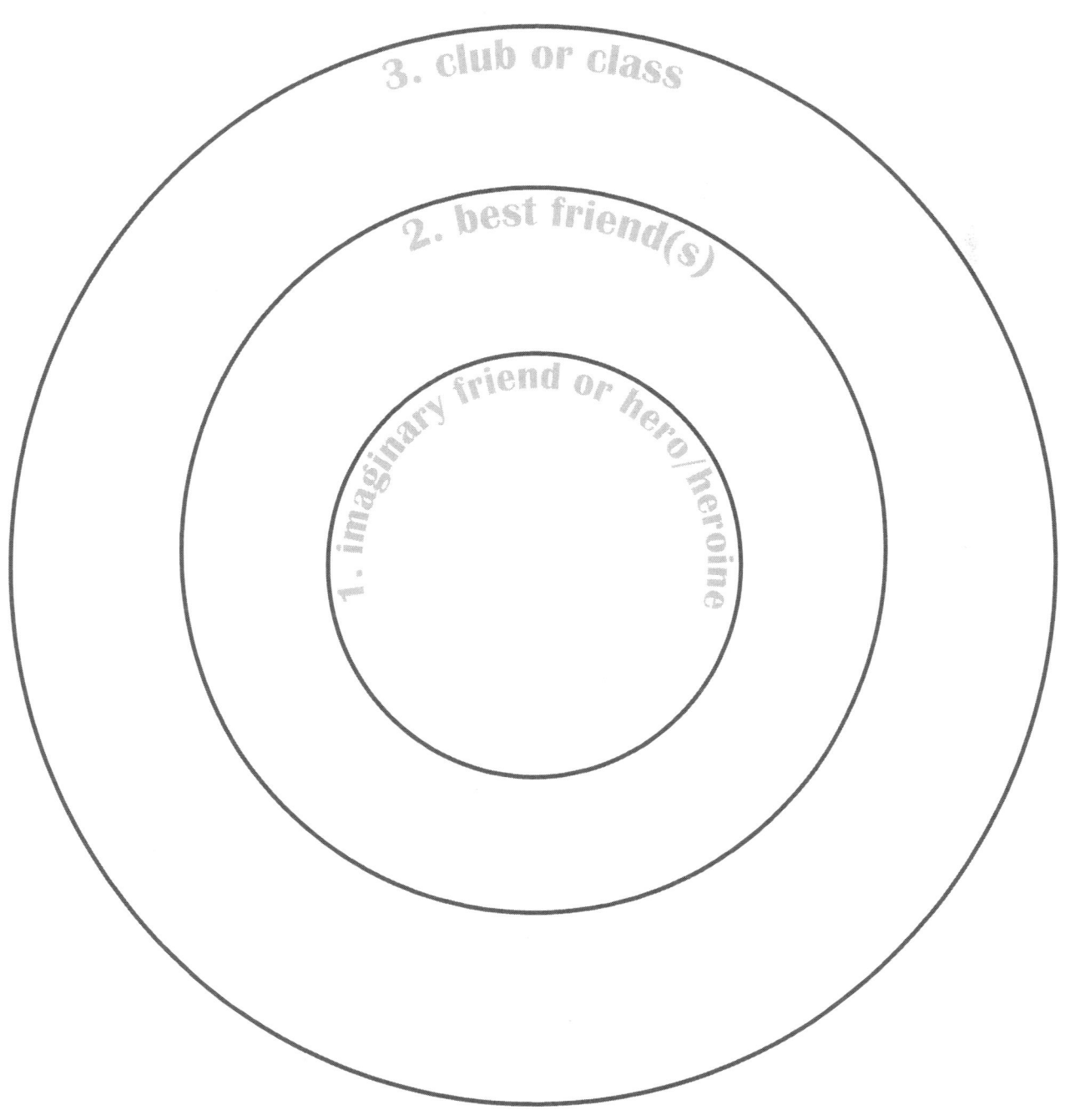

Worksheet 3e
Chains of Qualities & Strengths

One chain represents personal strengths and the second strengths and support from others. Colour and write in the two chains, see how they intertwine with each other.

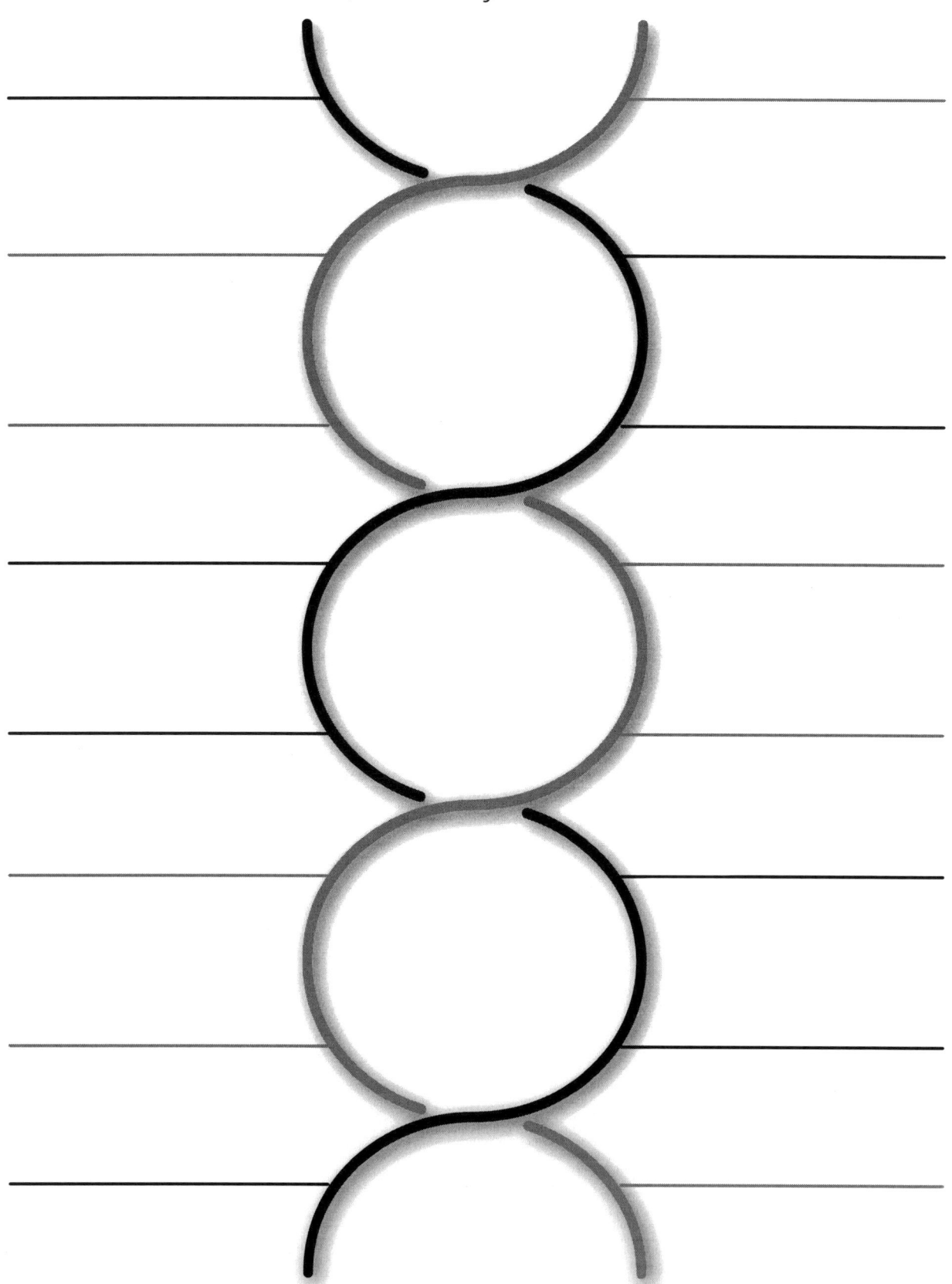

Section Four

Self-Soothing & Self-Care

Activities & Worksheets

Activities

4.1   Sensory, Rhythmic & Dramatic Activities

4.2   EPR Activities

4.3   Sensory Activities

Worksheets

4a   Hand Massage

4b   Special Scents & Smells

4c   Pleasant & Soothing Touch

4d   Special Food & Taste

4e   Special Sounds

Section Four

Self-Soothing & Self-Care

Trauma is experienced through all of the senses and throughout the body, and often the world no longer feels a safe place to be (see also Section Five The Safe Place). The senses are a reminder to people of many traumatic experiences: the smell of the fire, the sound of the roar of the sea, the taste of the polluted water, the touch of the paedophile, the sight of train crash. This sensory bombardment is so powerful that it can block out other sensory experiences, and people can have a strong reminder whenever they encounter a similar stimulus.

This section contains a range of sensory exercises from which teachers and therapists can select – carefully - depending on the experience and age-stage of their groups. The choice of activity should also be dependent on what the young people are ready for. For example, a child who has traumatised by touch will usually avoid all physical contact, but they can find massaging their own hands a soothing experience.

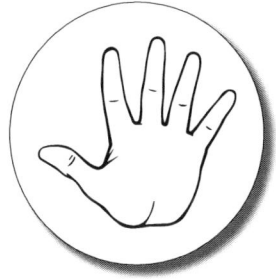

Please remember to use baby-oil, diluted essential oils, or a pink-coloured hand cream for massage, especially for children and teenagers who have been sexually abused. White hand-cream can have powerful associative memories.

The following three groups of activities are all variations on sensory activities. They need careful selection since people's experience will vary. However it important that a core of sensory work is completed before moving on to other sections (apart from Section Five The Safe Place).

Activities

All of the following techniques are suitable for Children and Teenagers.

Resources: Worksheets 4a to 4e, for selection where appropriate, essential oils, fleeces, calming posters for the walls, light-scented incense. Depending on the group's experiences, soothing music that is not associative (most CDs of Reiki music are very calming), sand trays and small toys if available, stories from Section Nine 'Healing Stories'.

Ambience: The room needs to be a nurturing space with a range of sensory choices, natural smells such as lavender or rosemary, rose petals, incense (be sure not to use artificial smells such as air fresheners, and some pot-pourri, as they are a source of many allergies, asthma, and eczema), comfortable cushions and large soft toys, with the possibility of snacks such as fresh fruit, and drinks if possible.

Explanation: Discuss with group members how many scary experiences can leave us feeling tense or anxious, and that it is important to re-discover some positive experiences, and that we can choose to explore different materials to help with this. In this group no-one will be forced to do any exercise. Everyone can explore the room and see what is there, and ask to have anything removed that they find unpleasant, and ask for other things to be included if it is possible. The following activities are all Neuro-Dramatic-Play (NDP), as described in the Introduction, and are intended to allow people to rediscover their early sensory experiences. Sensory, rhythmic and dramatic play (NDP) can help transform embedded trauma symptoms into playful and creative activity.

4.1 Sensory, Rhymthic & Dramatic Activities

Select ideas from the list below that are appropriate for the group at their stage of development. Spread them over several weeks and repeat any technique that is enjoyable. Keep the techniques as simple as possible, and allow them to be experienced in a calm atmosphere, with music if appropriate. For many of the techniques, it is possible to be wrapped up in a fleece and sit or lean on a cushion.

   i   Self-soothing through gentle massage, soothing warm drinks such as hot chocolate, calming stories and music.

   ii Rhythmic play with chanting, drum beats, developing an awareness of heart beats and how heart beats can change.

   iii Breathing exercises to breathe in the calm and breathe out the stress.

   iv Singing and humming enable tensions to be changed, and to create new patterns.

   v   Singing games and drama help to re-programme thoughts and feelings.

   vi Dramatic play: stories from the 'Six Part Story Assessment' and fairy stories can be drawn and enacted.

Endings: Give everyone the opportunity to write in their notebooks, place any completed Worksheets in folders; finish each session with breathing exercises, relaxation under a fleecy blanket, and a calming story.

4.2 EPR Activities

These activities use the techniques of Embodiment-Projection-Role (EPR), described in the introduction. A larger space is required to enable people to move around.

i Movement techniques to move out of the trauma (Embodiment), need to be developed cautiously as many young people will have experienced bodily trauma: stretching the whole body and then curling up again; stretching and breathing deeply and then letting go.

ii Dance and movement to rhythmic music can help to re-programme the body's trauma responses.

iii Allow the young person to play freely in the sand tray; they may or may not play out the traumatic event. The important issue is to support them to create symbolic new endings through gradually dismantling the figures and smoothing over the sand. Teachers and group leaders need to be vigilant as individuals may disclose material that requires therapeutic referral. However, it is possible for children and young people to create new endings to their stories that will enable them to move forward.

iv Choose one of the stories from Section Nine and use it for a drama and enactment (Role); have pieces of cloth and lots of hats available as props.

v Create a new drama based on ideas from drama games and improvisation (see p.141).

Endings: Give everyone the opportunity to write in their notebooks, place any completed Worksheets in folders; finish each session with breathing exercises, relaxation under a fleecy blanket, and a calming story.

4.3 Sensory Activities

Select from the Worksheets 4a to 4e to explore many of the issues discussed above. For some people the Worksheets will give a more concrete way of working and are specific in their instructions.

4a Hand Massage

4b Special Scents & Smells

4c Pleasant & Soothing Touch

4d Special Food & Taste

4e Special Sounds

Endings: Give everyone the opportunity to write in their notebooks, place any completed Worksheets in folders; finish each session with breathing exercises, relaxation under a fleecy blanket, and a calming story.

(For more NDP and EPR exercises see appendices in Jennings 2011.)

Worksheet 4a
Hand Massage

Using a little hand cream or baby oil, slowly carry out the following sequence of movements:

1. Rub the hands together.
2. Wrap one hand round the other and massage.
3. Use thumb of one hand to massage palm of other hand, then change over.
4. Stroke the back of the hand towards the body.
5. With middle finger and thumb, massage round each wrist.

These movements can also be done with a partner.

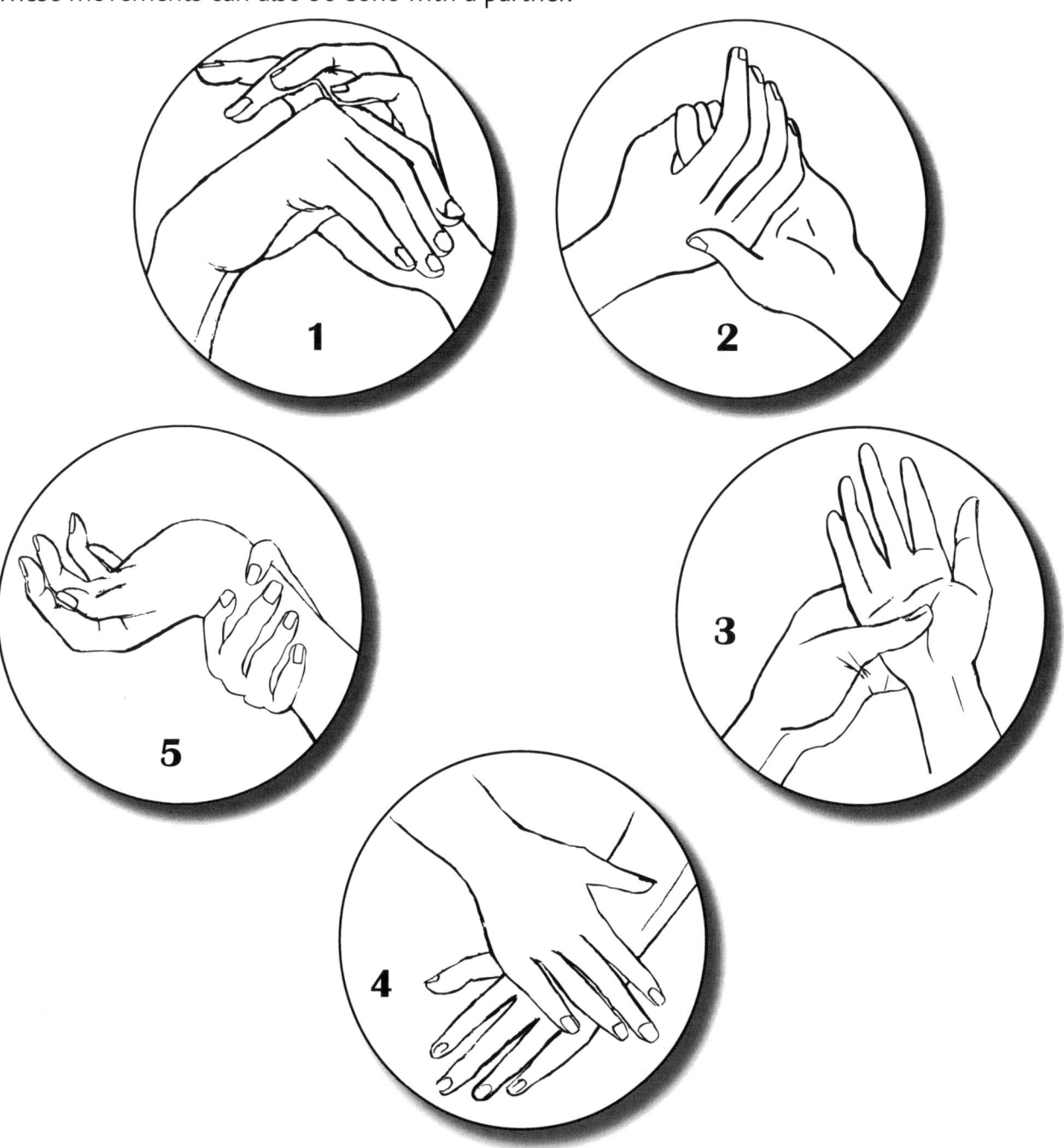

Worksheet 4b

Special Scents & Smells

Which of the following have smells that you like?

Colour in or write around the pictures what you like about them.

Choose any other smells you like and draw or write about them in the empty circles.

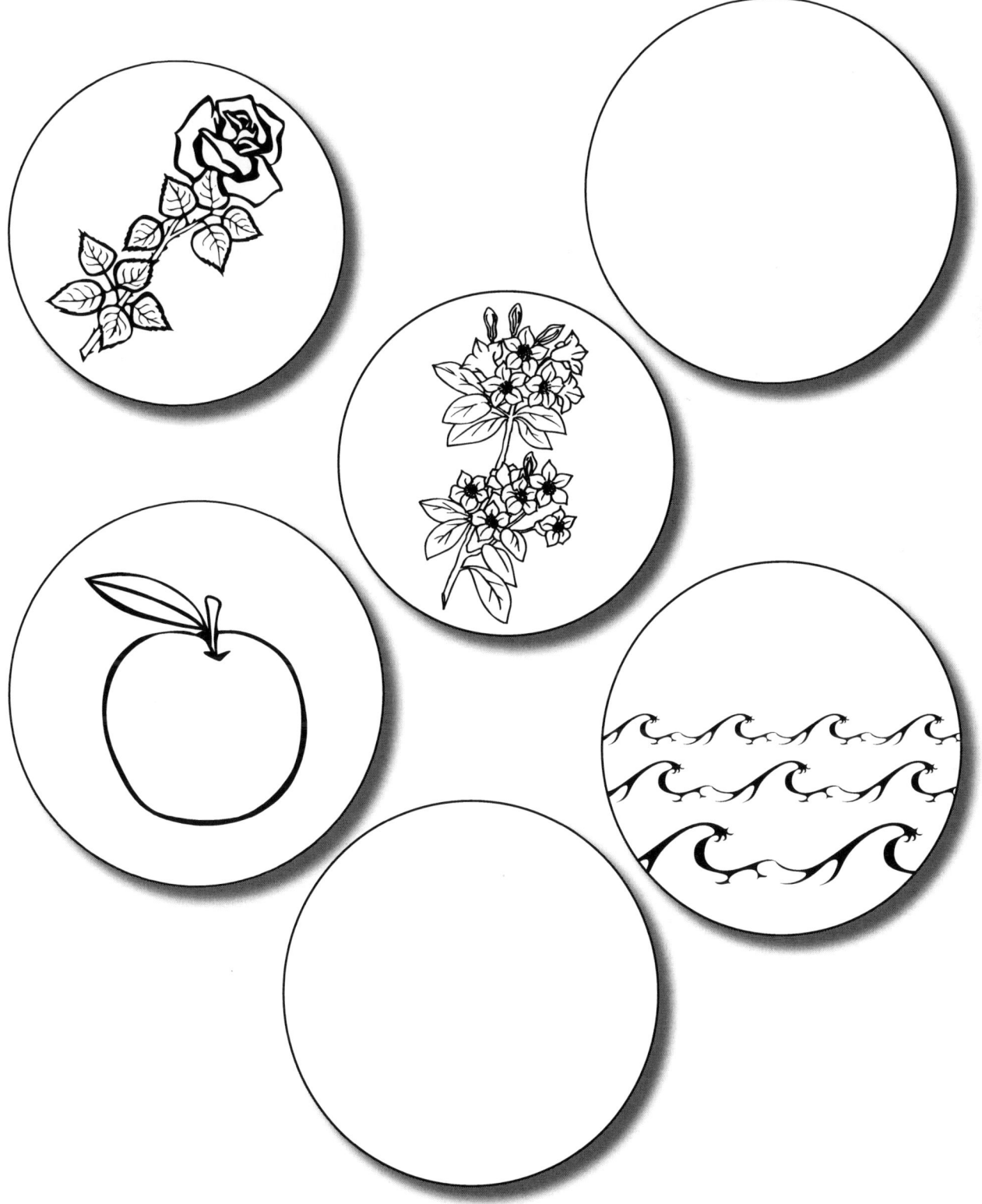

Worksheet 4c
Pleasant & Soothing Touch

As well as the touch from the hand massage, think about other touch that feels good.

Colour in the ones that are special for you.

Draw your own special touches that feel good.

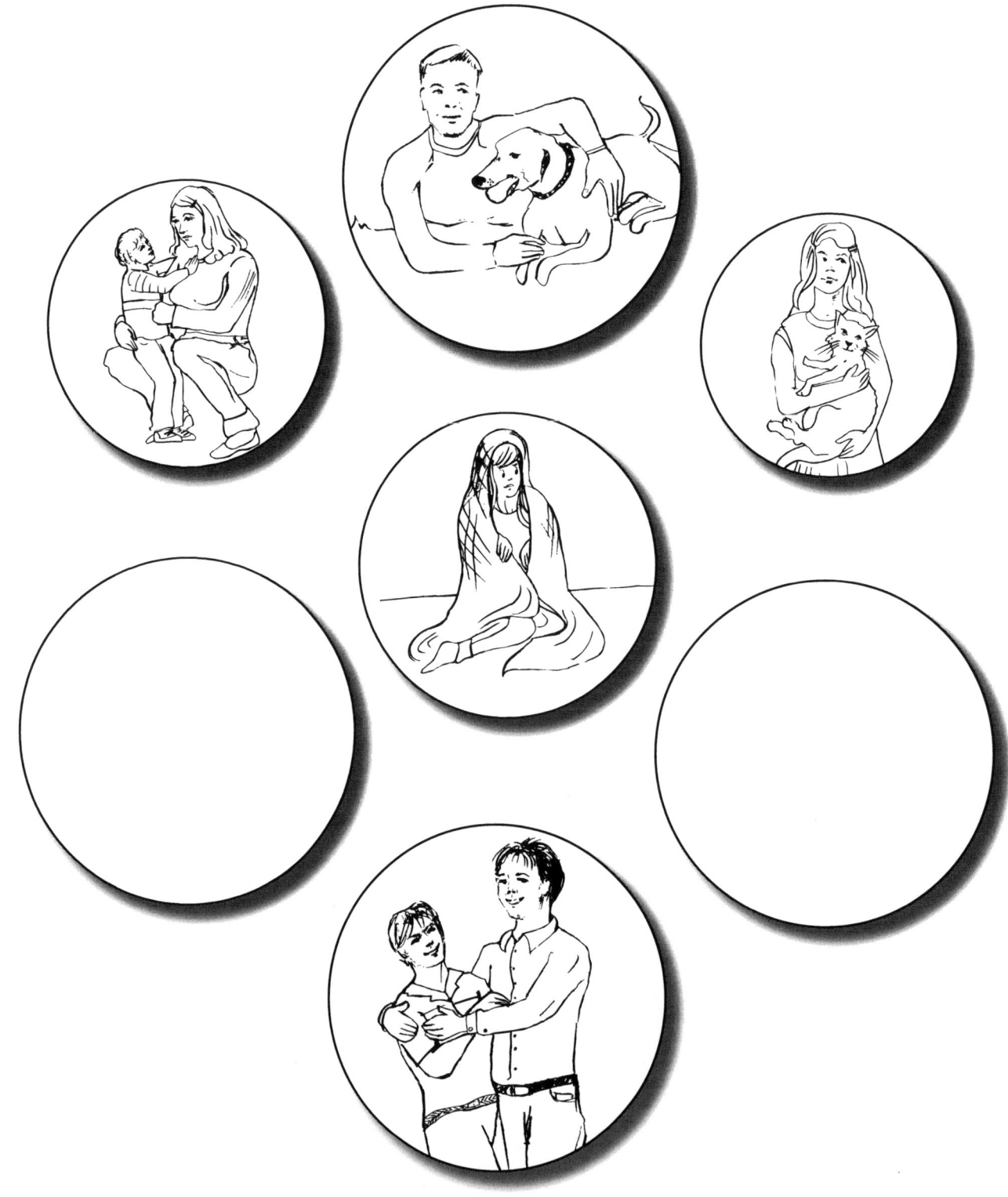

Worksheet 4d
Special Food & Taste

Think about food that tastes really great, and whether you can buy this food or whether someone makes it for you – or whether you can make it for yourself! Colour or write around the pictures of food that you really like.

Write about or draw your own pictures of special food and colour them.

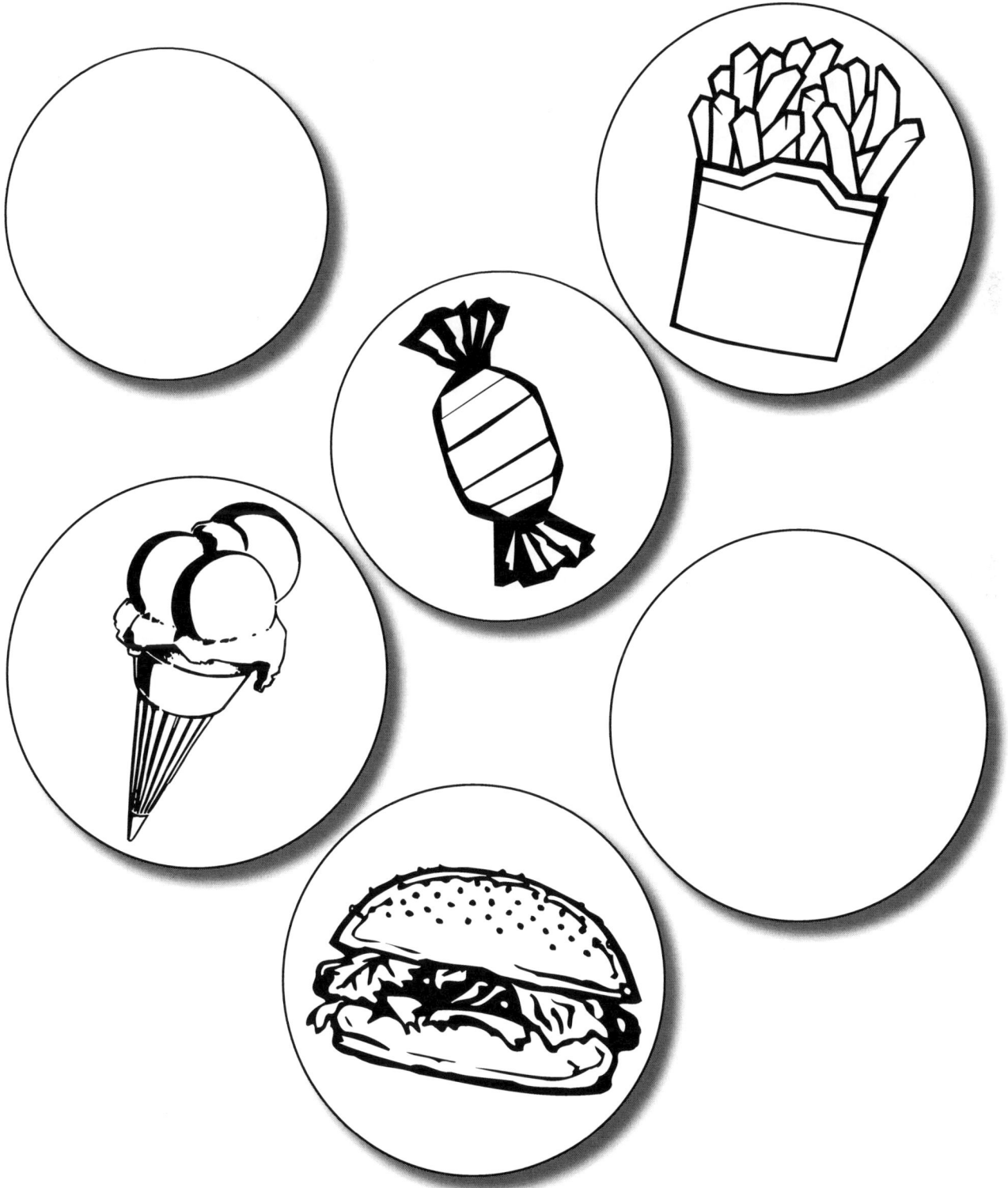

Worksheet 4e
Special Sounds

Think about all the different sounds that you enjoy: sounds outside such as birds singing, water running, or sounds you hear inside such as a cat purring or the music and songs that you like best.

Colour or write around the pictures of the sounds that you like.

Draw in the empty circles any other sounds that you really like.

Write down the names of your favourite music, bands and singers.

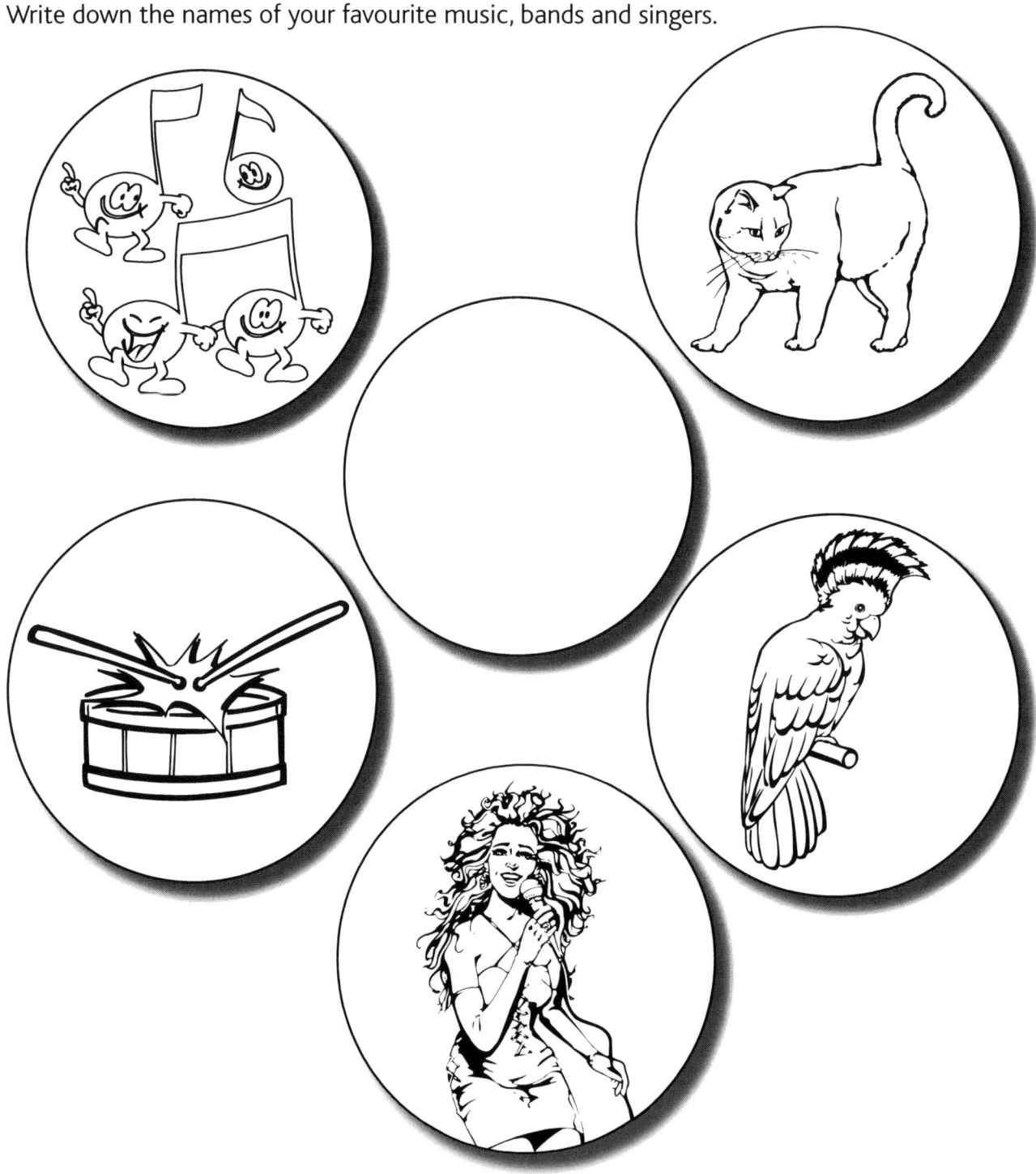

Section Five

The Safe Place

Activities & Worksheets

Activities

5.1 Creating a Safe Place
5.2 Feeling Safe

Worksheets

5a Where do I Feel Safe?
5b Where do I Not Feel Safe?
5c Safe Pictures in My Head
5d Scary Pictures in My Head
5e Creating a Safe Place

Section Five

The Safe Place

In order to carry out any trauma work it is essential to support the individual you are working with to create a safe place. They may build it in the therapy room (especially children) and then dismantle it at the end of the session, imagine it and draw it, or write a description of where it feels safe. For people who are still living in dangerous or fearful places, creative visualisation (described below) can be helpful as it allows them to have an image of their safe place in their mind. Safe places vary for everyone and it is important to remember that we cannot assume that a certain place is safe. For example, for the teenager who is suffering sexual abuse, their bedroom is not the safe place that it would be for many people.

Activities

Unless indicated all of the following exercises are suitable for both Children and Teenagers.

Resources: Large quantities of re-cycling materials, as varied as possible, for example: large boxes (e.g., from electrical goods), packaging from products, small boxes, old wool, string, shiny wrappers. Art materials: paper, clay or Plasticine, crayons, staplers, scissors, large pieces of cloth (not for cutting up), scraps of fabric, fleeces and stories from Section Nine.

Explanation: Introduce the idea of how important it is to keep ourselves safe, however old we are. It is important to imagine a place that feels safe, and to think about what is there as well as what must not be there. Everyone is going to have the opportunity to create their own 'safe place' with whatever materials they wish.

5.1 Creating a Safe Place

i Make use of the re-cycled materials and build a shelter that feels a special place: tables or chairs could be used as a frame or the large boxes; decorate it however you wish.

ii Everyone closes their eyes (or shades them if that is too scary) and imagines they are going on a walk to a safe place, somewhere in nature: how will you get there? Are there barriers to overcome? At last you get there and find your way inside. You stay for a few moments, making sure you can remember the place, then close the entrance and make your way back again. You are here in the room with everyone else. Draw and colour the safe place you have discovered.

iii Repeat the same instructions, and create the journey to the safe place and back again; after opening eyes, invite everyone to create a model of their safe place using the recycled materials.

iv Repeat the same instructions, and create the journey to the safe place and back again; after opening eyes, invite everyone to make a model of their safe place from clay or Plasticine.

v Invite everyone to think about whether it is more important to have doors open for escape or doors closed to protect in their safe place. Draw a picture of a safe place and indicate the doors.

Endings: Give everyone the opportunity to write in their notebook and to place any completed Worksheets into folder; finish each session with breathing exercises, relaxation under a fleecy blanket, and a calming story (See Section Nine).

5.2 Feeling Safe

Use Worksheets 5a to 5e to explore many of the issues discussed above. For some people the Worksheets provide a more concrete way of working and are specific in their instructions. The Worksheets also suggest possible safe/unsafe places that people may not have considered before.

5a Where do I Feel Safe?

5b Where do I Not Feel Safe?

5c Safe Pictures in My Head

5d Scary Pictures in My Head

5e Creating a Safe Place

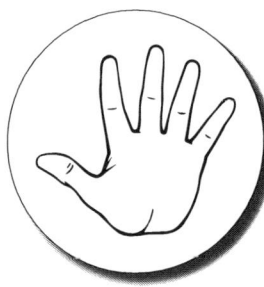

Some people may not be ready for Worksheets 5b and 5d and these must be introduced with care. It may be necessary to build up a lot more strengths around safe places (Worksheet 5e can be helpful in this respect), through drawing or modelling or building, before introducing the unsafe ones. However, some individuals may bring up the topic themselves and be happy to explore it. One child built a safe shelter inside a wall surrounded by guards for ten weeks before feeling safe to move on.

Endings: Give everyone the opportunity to write in their notebook and to place any completed Worksheets into folder; finish each session with breathing exercises, relaxation under a fleecy blanket, and a calming story (See Section Nine).

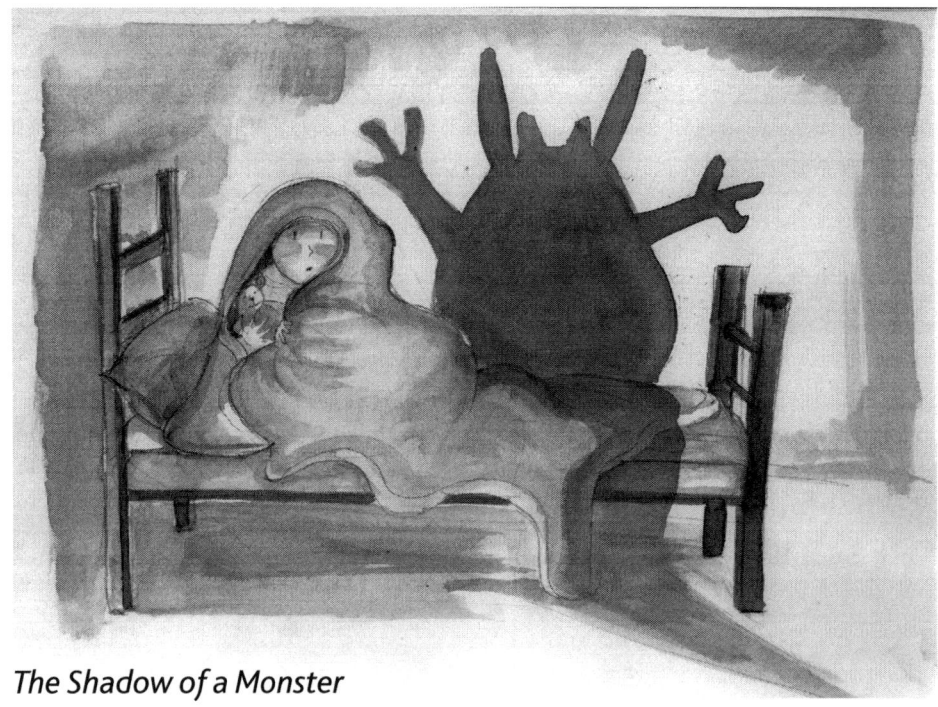

The Shadow of a Monster

Worksheet 5a

Where do I Feel Safe?

There are different places where people feel safe, some are indoors and some are outdoors. Colour the places where you feel safe and write or draw your own ideas as well.

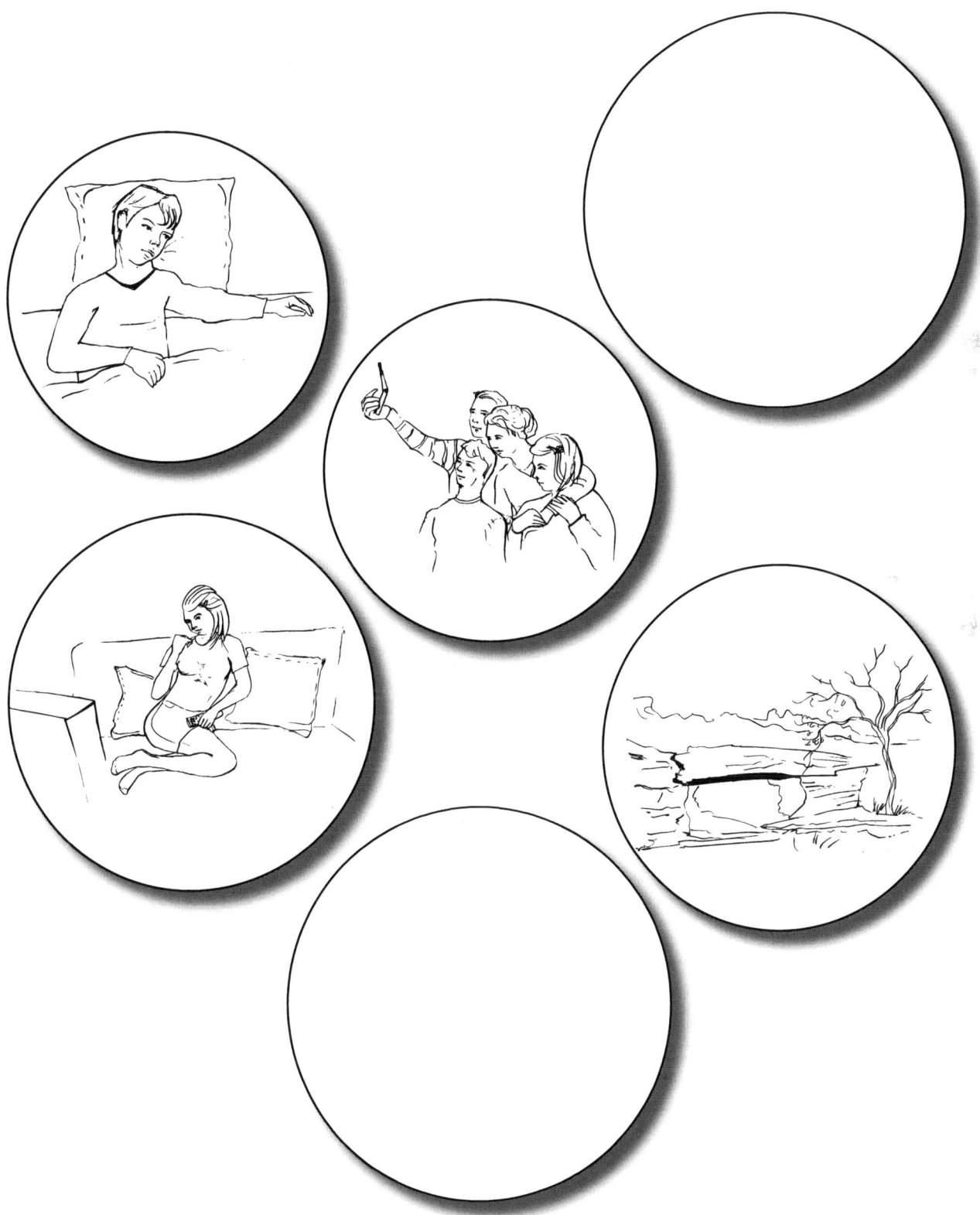

Worksheet 5b

Where do I Not Feel Safe?

Think of places that feel scary and where you don't feel safe.

Maybe they are real places or they could be places that you think could be scary.

Draw or write about any place where you don't feel safe or that feels scary.

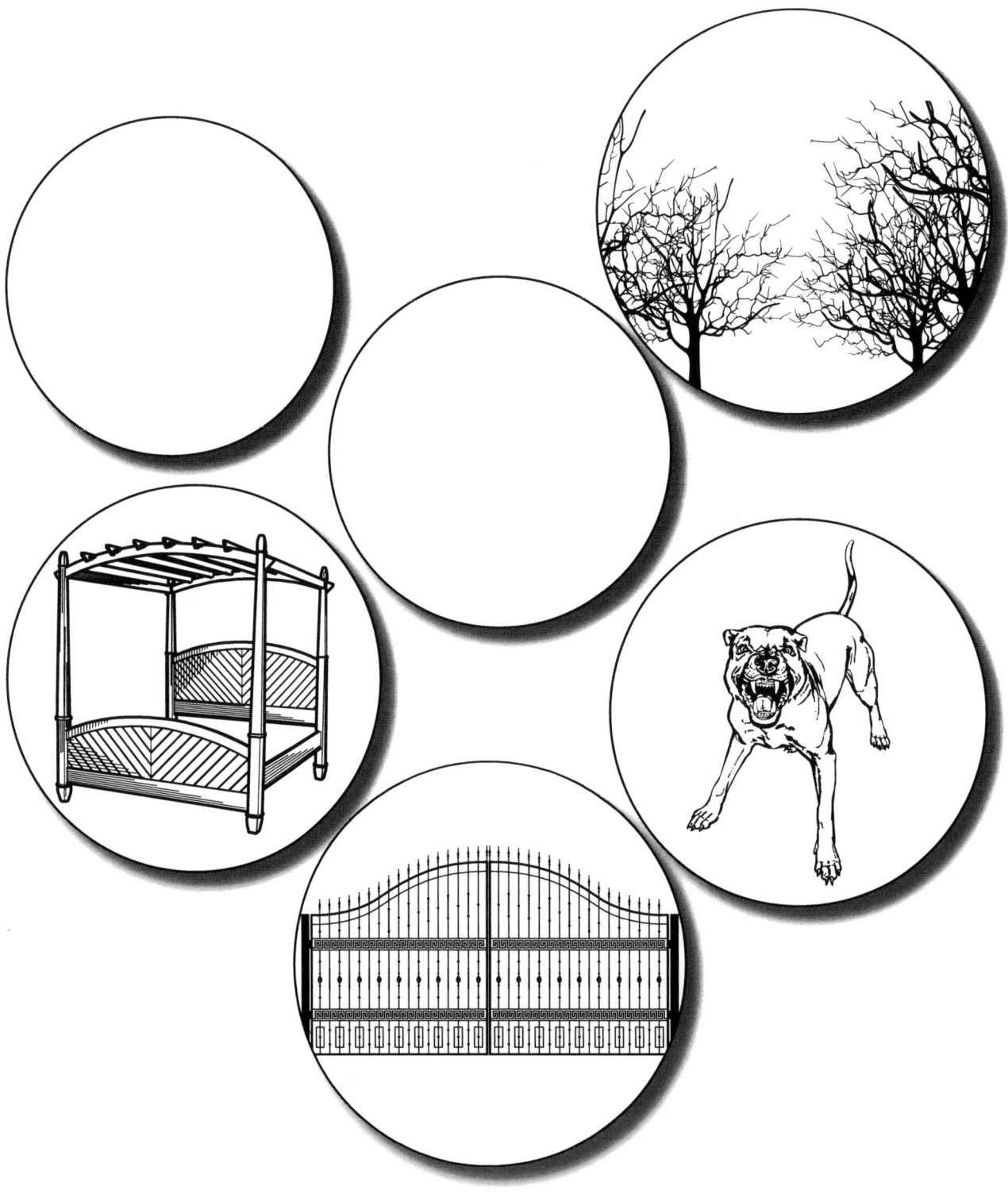

56   This page may be photocopied for instructional use only. *When the World Falls Apart* © Sue Jennings 2015

Worksheet 5c

Safe Pictures in my Head

It is important to have pictures in your head that feel safe and secure, and then to be able to think of them in scary or unsafe moments. Colour any pictures that feel safe. Colour or write safe words that you can keep in your head.

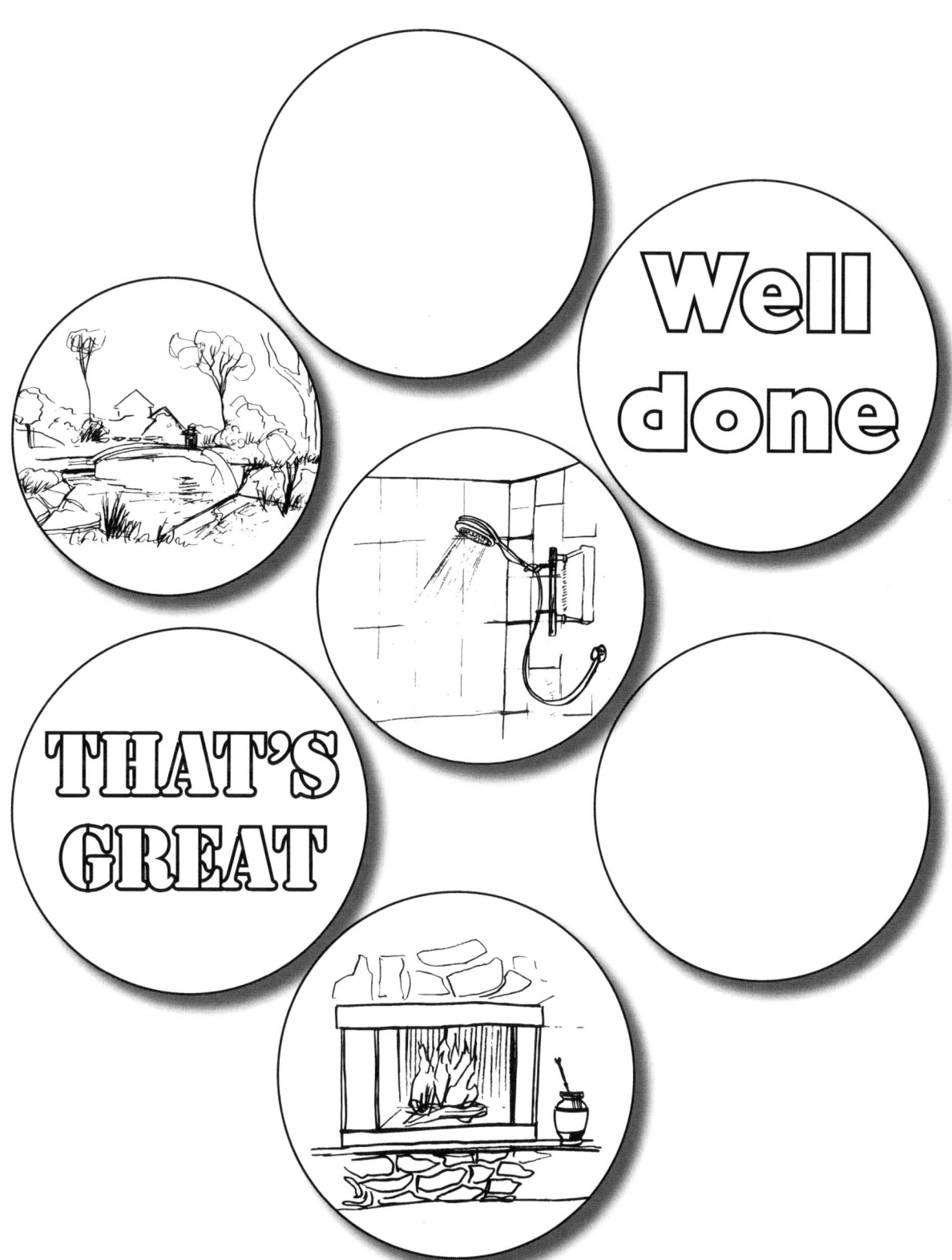

Worksheet 5d
Scary Pictures in My Head

Often scary pictures stay in our heads after a frightening experience. Sometimes it helps to name these pictures so that we can control them. Colour any pictures that feel scary for you and also create your own if you wish.

Draw or write about your own pictures that stay in your head.

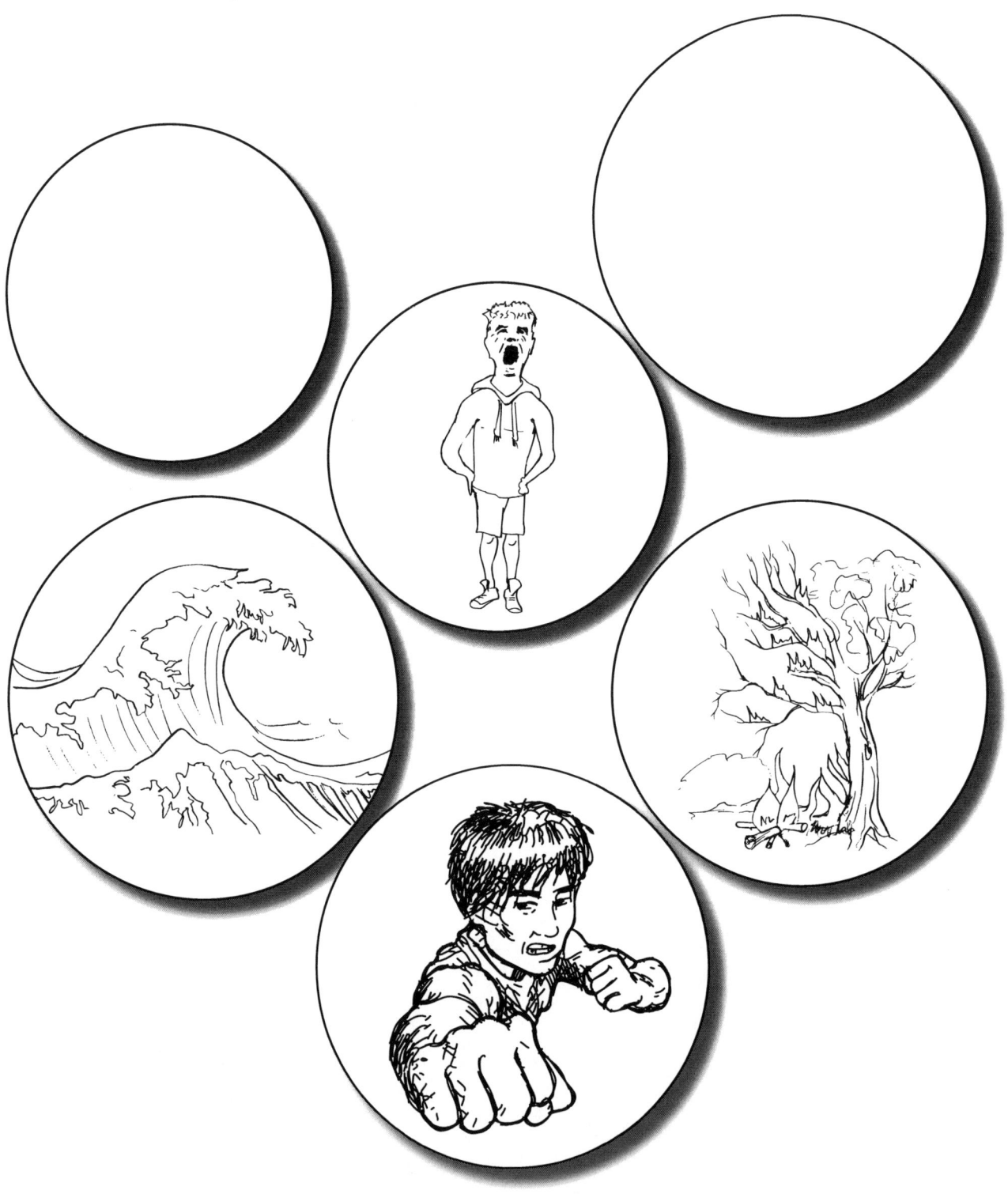

Worksheet 5e
Creating a Safe Place

Think of a space that you can create that would have everything in it to feel safe. What would it be made of? Wood? Bricks? What colour would it be? Would it have any notices outside (perhaps 'Keep Out!')? Draw your own safe place showing what is inside and outside and colour it in.

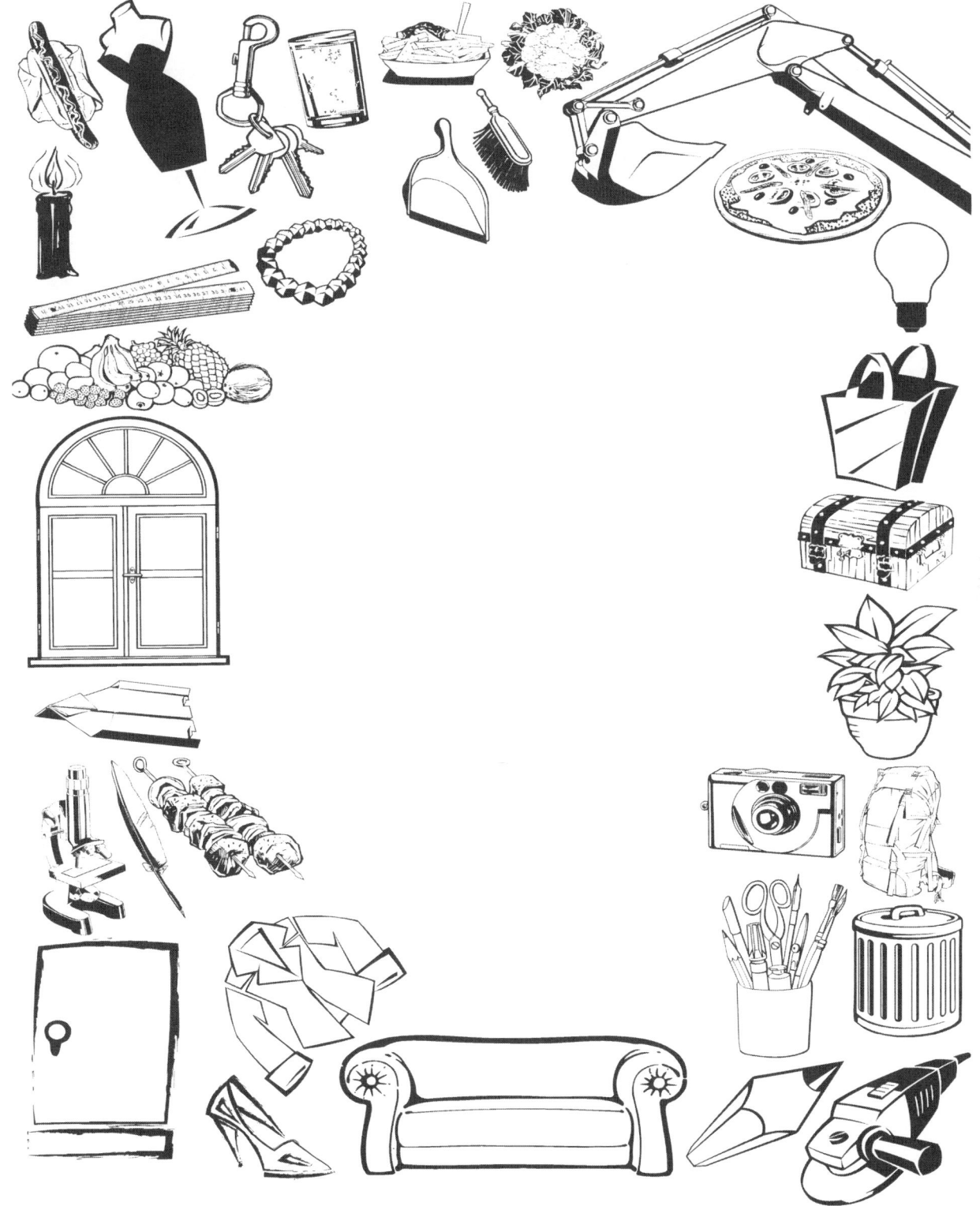

Section Six

Night Fears & Nightmares

Activities & Worksheets

Activities

6.1 Neuro-Dramatic Play
6.2 Worksheet Activities

Worksheets

6a When it Gets Dark ... the Scary Moments
6b When it Gets Dark ... the Good Moments
6c How Can Other People Help?
6d How Can I Help Myself?
6e Waking Up Nightmares

Section Six

Night Fears & Nightmares

For many children and teenagers, the night is a very scary time, especially when it gets dark early, if bedroom doors are shut and if there are no lights apart from those that cause shadow. If children are scared, it does not help to 'toughen them up' and leave them in the dark. For children and teenagers who have been traumatised, the experience is even worse and great care needs to be given to the ambience of their bedroom. When young people are recovering from trauma it may be that a night light is needed, the bedroom door left open, a landing or lavatory light left on, and a warm dressing gown and slippers left by the bed. There is no doubt that a relaxing, sensory bath (using for instance, candles, special bubble-bath, gentle incense, warm towels) can be helpful before bedtime; providing of course someone has not been traumatised by water. By finishing these sessions with a 'bedtime story', while relaxing with the fleece, you are creating a role-model that perhaps could be followed up at home.

Activities

Unless indicated all of the following exercises are suitable for both Children and Teenagers.

Resources: Worksheets 6a to 6e, for selection where appropriate depending on the experiences of the group, soothing music that is not associative, notebooks, folders, fleeces. Most CDs of Reiki music are very calming, stories from Section Nine Healing Stories.

Ambience: The room needs to be a nurturing space with a range of sensory choices, natural smells such as lavender or rosemary, rose petals, incense (be sure not to use artificial smells such as air fresheners, and some pot-pourri, as they are a source of many allergies, asthma, and eczema), comfortable cushions and large soft toys, with the possibility of snacks such as fresh fruit, and drinks if possible.

Explanation: Discuss with group members how many scary experiences take place at night, leaving us feeling tense or anxious, unable to sleep or experiencing nightmares. It is important to rediscover some positive experiences in order to change our night routine. Children and teenagers can be encouraged to share some of the techniques they learn with parents or carers when at home and to see if parental support could allow their bedtime routine to change. The following activities are all Neuro-Dramatic-Play (as outlined in the Introduction) and are intended to allow people to rediscover safe-sleeping. Sensory, Rhythmic and Dramatic Play (NDP) can help to change embedded trauma symptoms into playful and creative activity.

6.1 Neuro-Dramatic-Play

   i   Play a ball game where everyone says their name as the ball is thrown (be careful with individuals who are not well coordinated and could easily drop the ball).

   ii Hold hands with a partner and skip, hop and jump together or with teenagers, try to run a 3-legged race, without an ankle tie (avoid this activity if the young people are wary of touch or use a hoop or length of fabric to 'connect).

   iii With a partner, take it in turns to play percussion (gently) on each other's backs (wrap in fleeces if sensitive to touch).

   iv With a partner share a positive picture that can be imagined at bedtime in order to help go to sleep.

   v   Sit wrapped up in fleeces and practice deep breathing.

6.2 Worksheet Activities

Use Worksheets 6a to 6e to explore many of the issues discussed above. For some people the Worksheets provide a more concrete way of working and are specific in their instructions. The Worksheets also suggest new ways to approach safe sleep that perhaps have not been considered before.

6a When it Gets Dark ... the Scary Moments

6b When it Gets Dark ... the Good Moments

6c How Can Other People Help?

6d How Can I Help Myself?

6e Waking up Nightmares

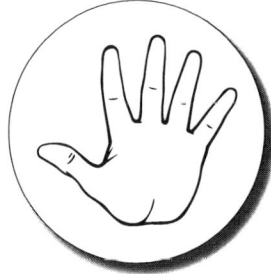

You should exercise caution with using Worksheet 6a, but it may well be that members of the group have by now done enough work to cope with this Worksheet.

Endings: Give everyone the opportunity to write or draw in their notebooks and place any completed worksheets into folders; finish each session with breathing exercises, relaxation under a fleecy blanket and a calming story (see Section Nine).

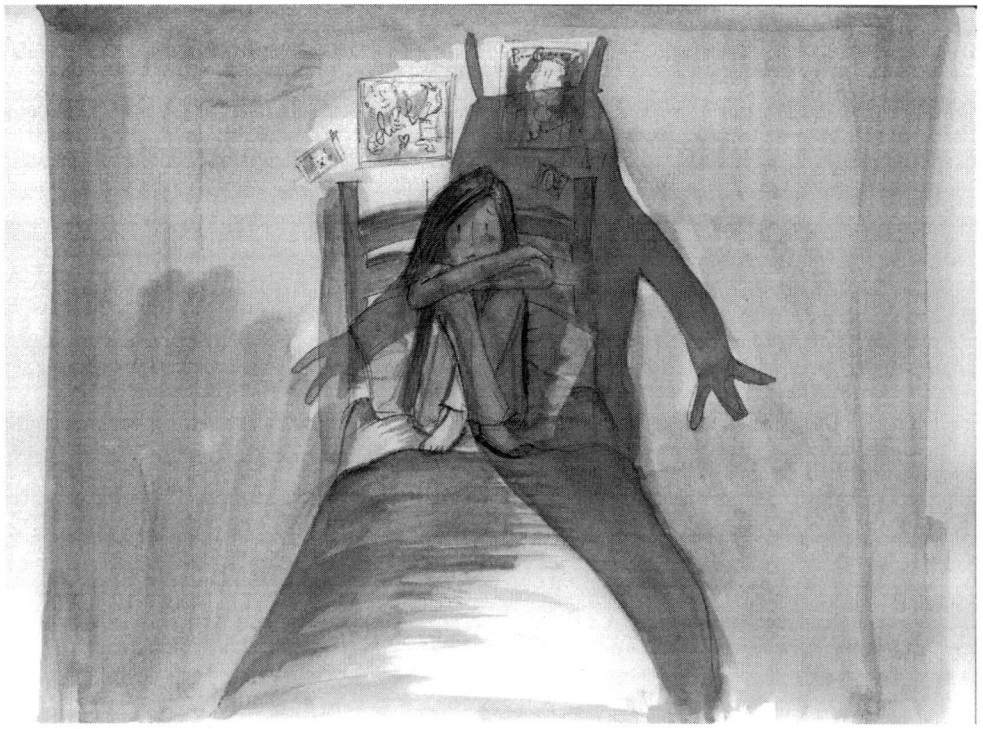

Night Fears and Nightmares

Worksheet 6a

When it Gets Dark... the Scary Moments

When the sun goes down or the lights are turned off it can feel a very scary place.

What are the thoughts and pictures that come to mind when it is dark?

Is it sounds that you can hear, or do you see pictures in your head or shadows on the wall?

Write or draw the scary moments in the circles below; you can use words or pictures or both.

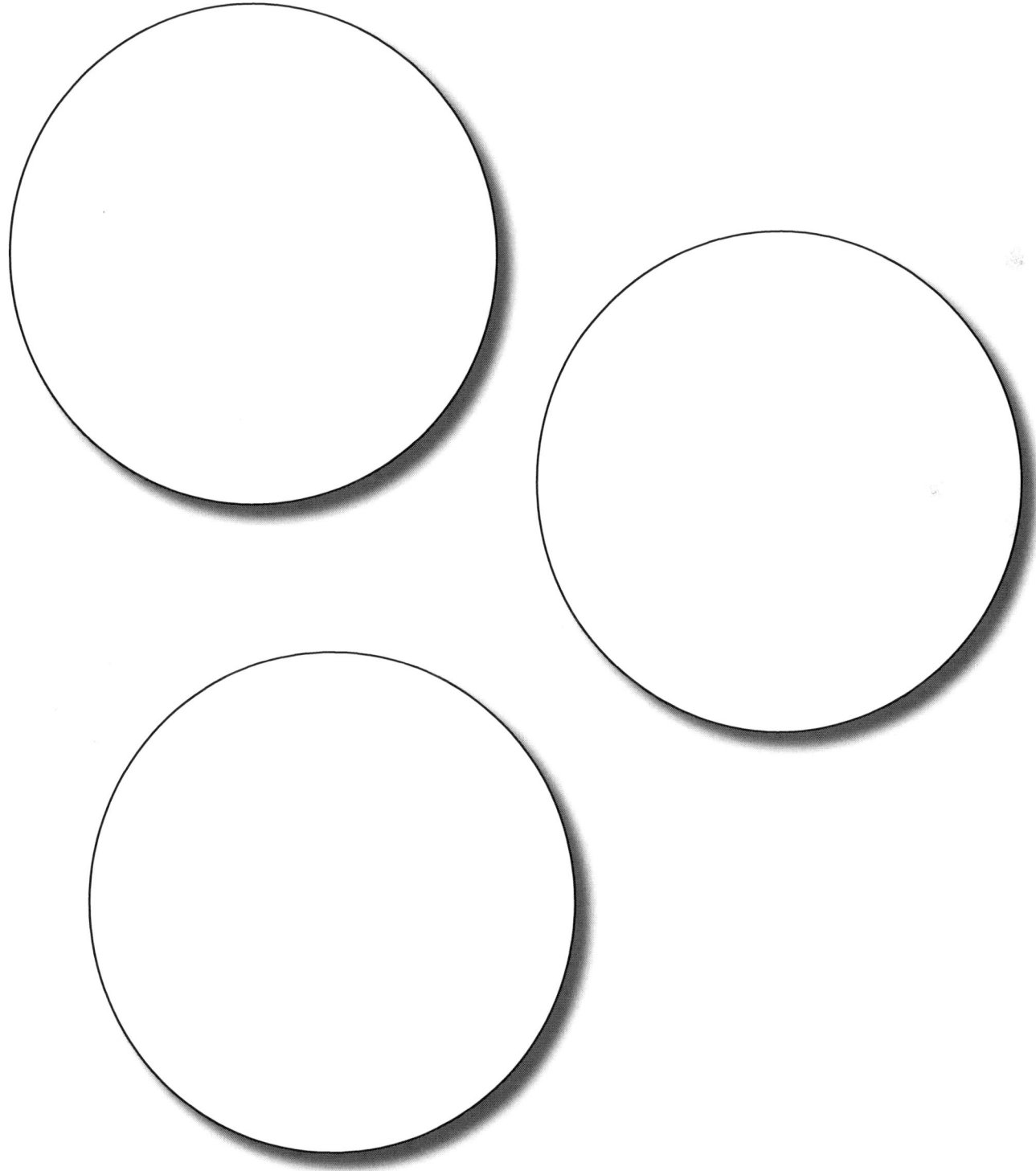

Worksheet 6b

When it Gets Dark... the Good Moments

When the dark feels scary it can sometimes help to think about positive times and to create positive pictures in our heads. These could be things that have happened that you enjoyed, or when you felt good because someone liked something you did or when you found a new special friend.

Think about several things that make you feel good inside and create the pictures in your head. Then draw them or write about them in the circles.

You can draw pictures or write about them or do both.

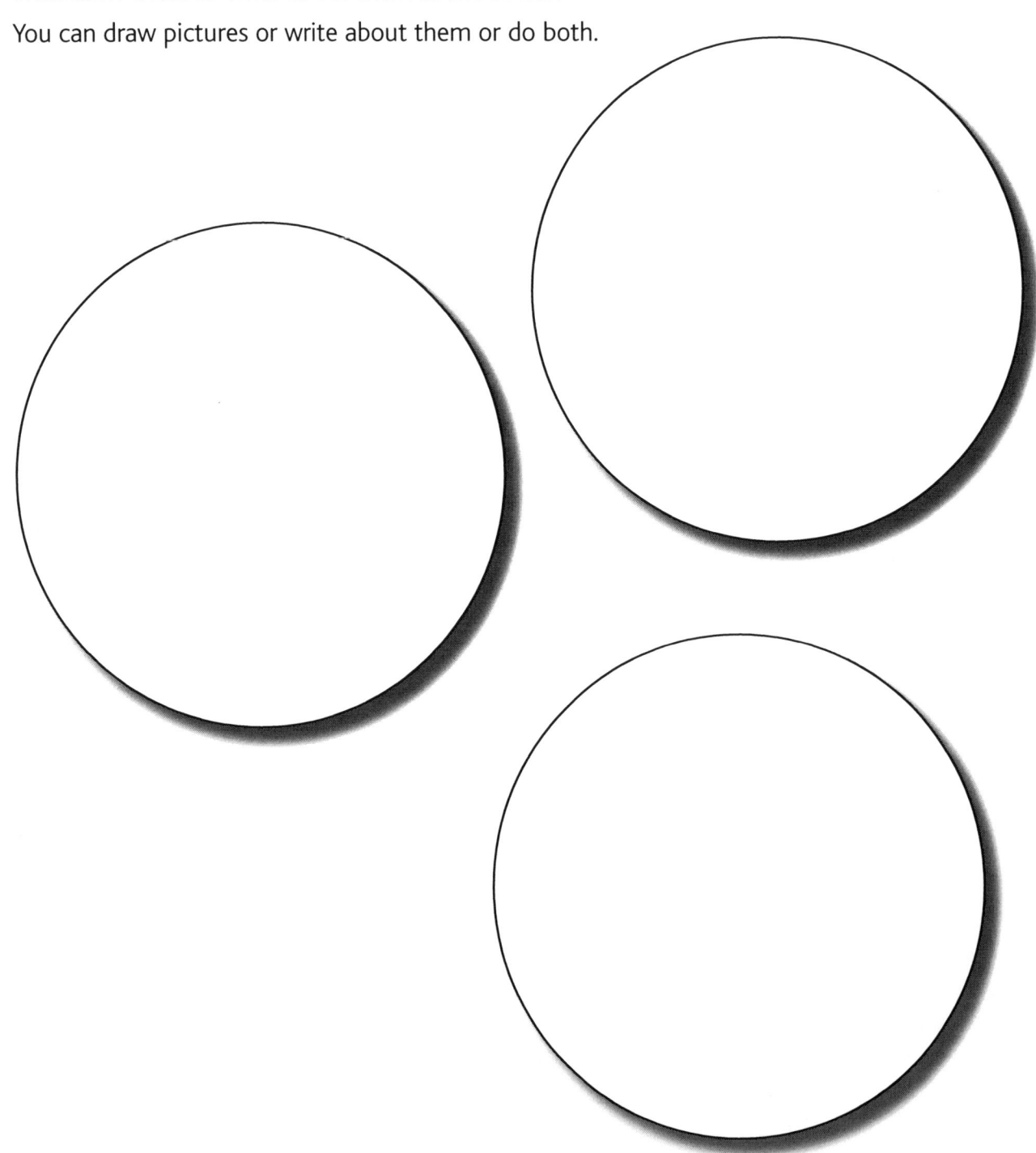

Worksheet 6c

How Can Other People Help?

Often there are simple things that other people can do to help us feel calm and safe. For example, many people do not like the dark so perhaps someone could get you a night light or leave the landing light on and leave the bedroom door open.

Sometimes having a new cosy bed cover helps because it can help make bed feel like a nest. Perhaps being made a hot milky drink with honey can help at bedtime.

Think about what other people might do to help you feel safe at night, especially when it is very dark. Draw or write about these things in the circles below.

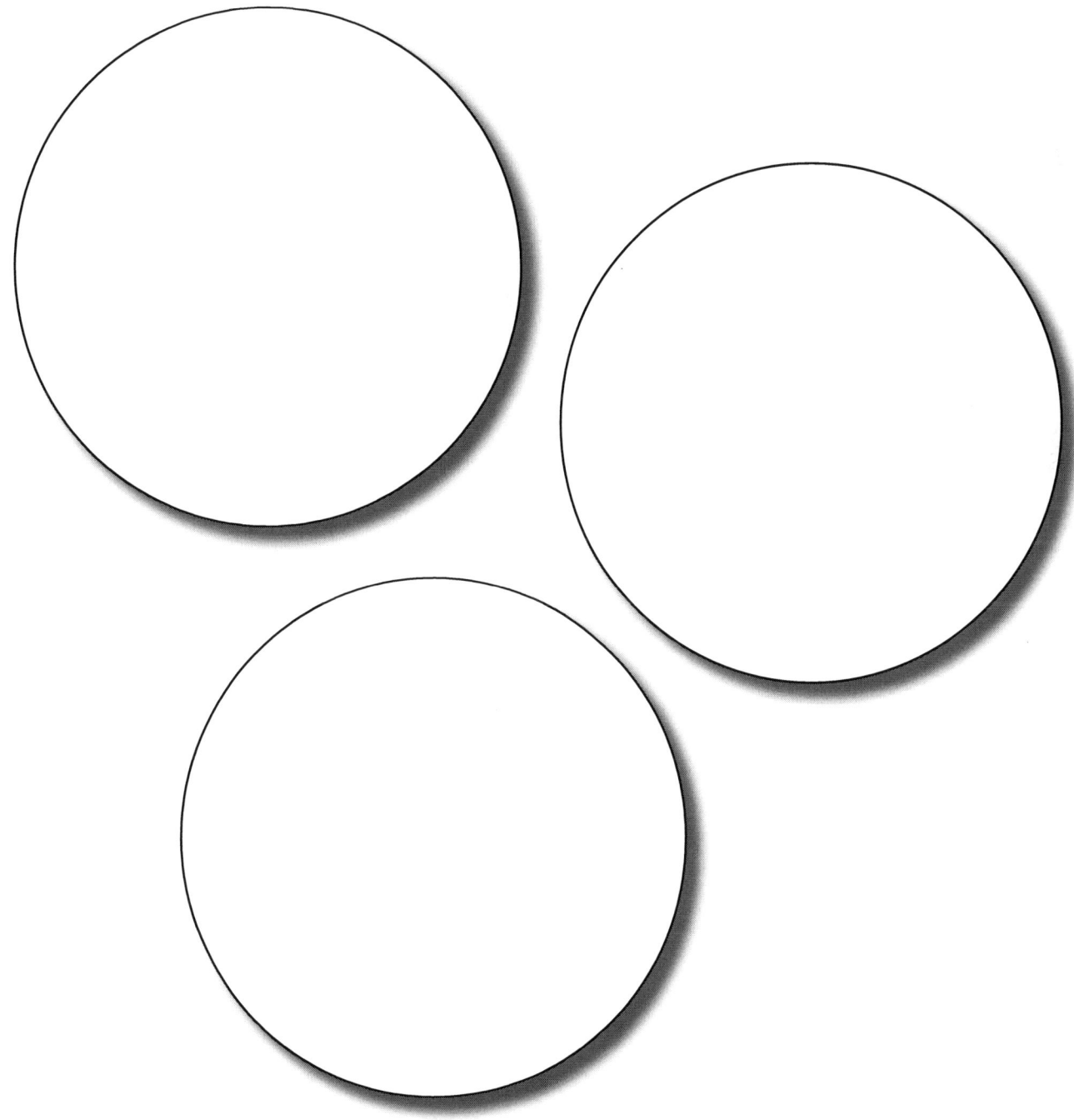

This page may be photocopied for instructional use only. *When the World Falls Apart* © Sue Jennings 2015

Worksheet 6d

How Can I Help Myself?

Think about some simple things that you might do to stay calm at night. There could be the things that you can ask other people from the last Worksheet to do, but perhaps you could do some of them for yourself. Do you still have a toy that you had when you were little? A teddy or cuddly rabbit, perhaps. Sometimes these special toys can be helpful when we are scared, however old we are! Many grown-ups still have their cuddly toysd and sit it on their beds. There are other things you can do such as leaving the curtains open just a little so some light from the moon or street lights can shine in. Watching scary stuff on TV or online does not help us relax at bedtime. Think about having a warm shower or bath with nice soap or bath gel before you go to bed.

Draw or write three things you could do to help yourself stay calm and relaxed at bedtime.

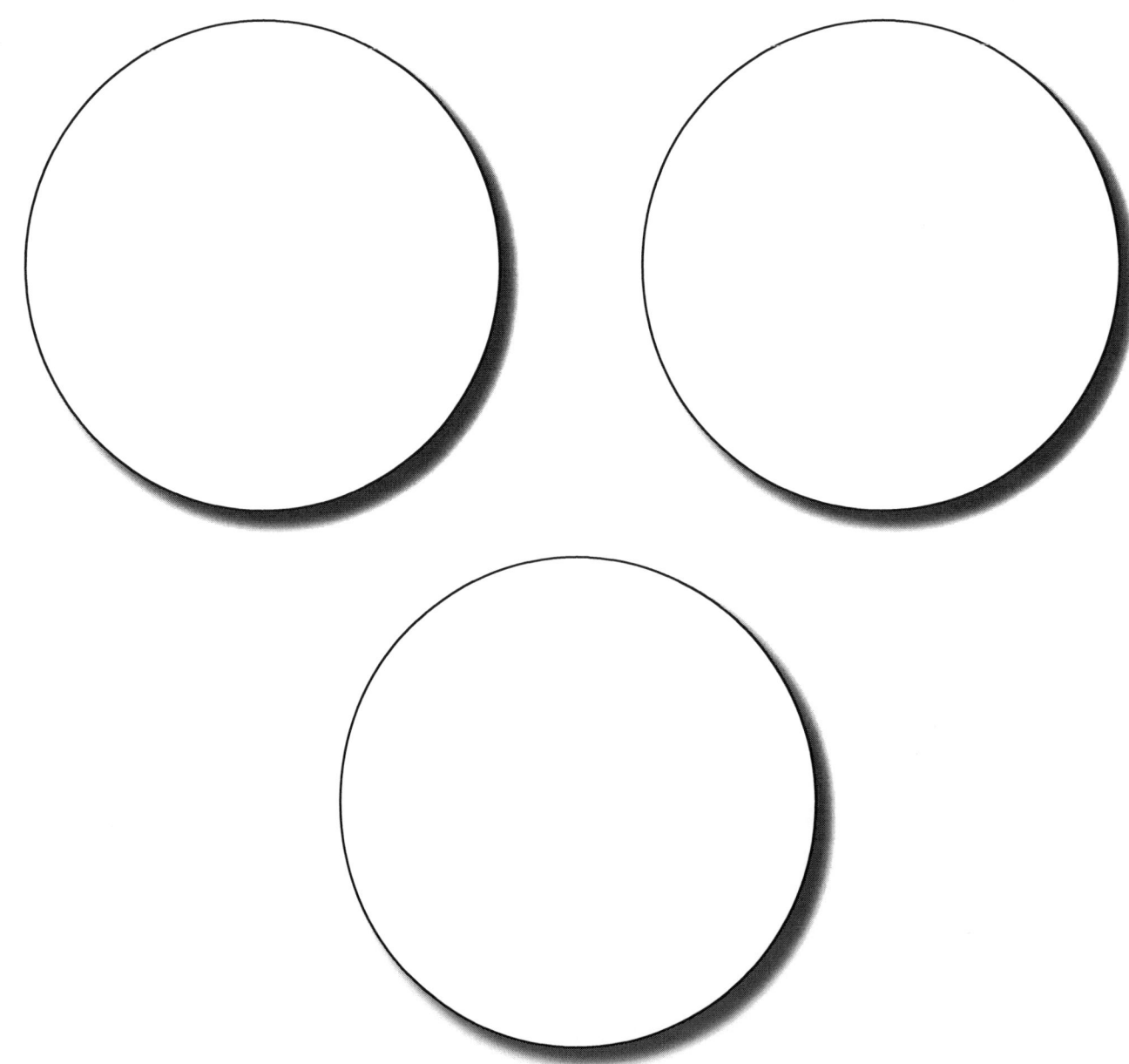

Worksheet 6e
Waking Up Nightmares

Sometimes even if we manage to go to sleep calmly, we might wake up from a frightening dream and may see or hear or smell frightening memories. These can seem less frightening if we have a night light in the room or if we can see light outside the window. However, it is very scary and often we might sweat or panic breathe or feel our heart racing.

The following exercises can help:

1. Sit up in bed or the chair and breath deeply: slowly in and slowly out.
   (There are examples of more breathing exercises in Section Three).
2. Stretch your whole body from top to toe and give a big yawn lying down or standing.
3. Take time to read your favourite book or comic before falling asleep again.
4. Think about the things that you are looking forward to doing tomorrow.
5. Think about something really silly or a joke that will make you smile or laugh.

Can you think of other things you might do to help you settle down again? Write or draw the things that might help you with your nightmares.

_____

_____

_____

This page may be photocopied for instructional use only. *When the World Falls Apart* © Sue Jennings 2015

Section Seven

Challenging the Monsters

Activities & Worksheets

Activities

7.1   EPR Activities
7.2   Worksheet Activities

Worksheets

7a   Monsters in the Shadows
7b   How I Feel Inside
7c   Challenging the Monster
7d   Scary Spaces & Places
7e   Talking to the Dream Monster
7f   The Story of My Monster
7g   Scary Shadows
7h   Monster Under the Bed
7i   Meeting & Welcoming the Monster

Section Seven

Challenging the Monsters

Many children and young people who have been traumatised perceive the bully or the abuser or the institution as monstrous. Monsters seem to be so powerful that their victims can only freeze or flee rather than fight or protest. McCarthy (2012) suggests that we need to be aware that many children are helped by drawing themselves as a monster – as one who has power -and to allow it to be alive in the play room. He invites children at the beginning of therapy to draw themselves 'as if' they are a monster (also McCarthy 2007). The making of the image of the monster, whether it is the self or other, enables the child to gain mastery over the monster: whether it is empowering them to be monstrous or conquering the monstrous abuser. It is important that we work with 'the monster', whether internal or external so that we can work without the blame, shame and guilt that sabotage , trauma work. They are all part of the destructive qualities of the monster.

Challenging the Monsters

Activities

All of the following exercises are suitable for both Children and Teenagers.

Resources: Worksheets 7a to 7i, for selection where appropriate, depending on the experiences of the group, lots of old newspapers, masking tape, paper, coloured pens, clay or Plasticine, notebooks and folders, soothing music that is not associative. Most CDs of Reiki music are very calming, fleeces, stories from Section Nine Healing Stories.

Ambience: The room needs to be a nurturing space with a range of sensory choices, natural smells such as lavender or rosemary (be sure not to use artificial smells such as air fresheners, and some pot-pourri, as they can be a source of many allergies, asthma, and eczema), there needs to be room to move about, with the possibility of snacks such as fresh fruit, and drinks if possible.

Explanation: Discuss with group members how many scary experiences can be like monsters, or they can feel like something unknown and very scary that is coming to get us. Maybe these monster-like feelings keep us awake at night (see Section Six) or maybe they leave us feeling tense or anxious, and sometimes we feel physically ill. It is important to rediscover some positive experiences to change our monster ways of thinking, and then perhaps we can make friends with our monster as in the 'Greeting the Monster' picture.

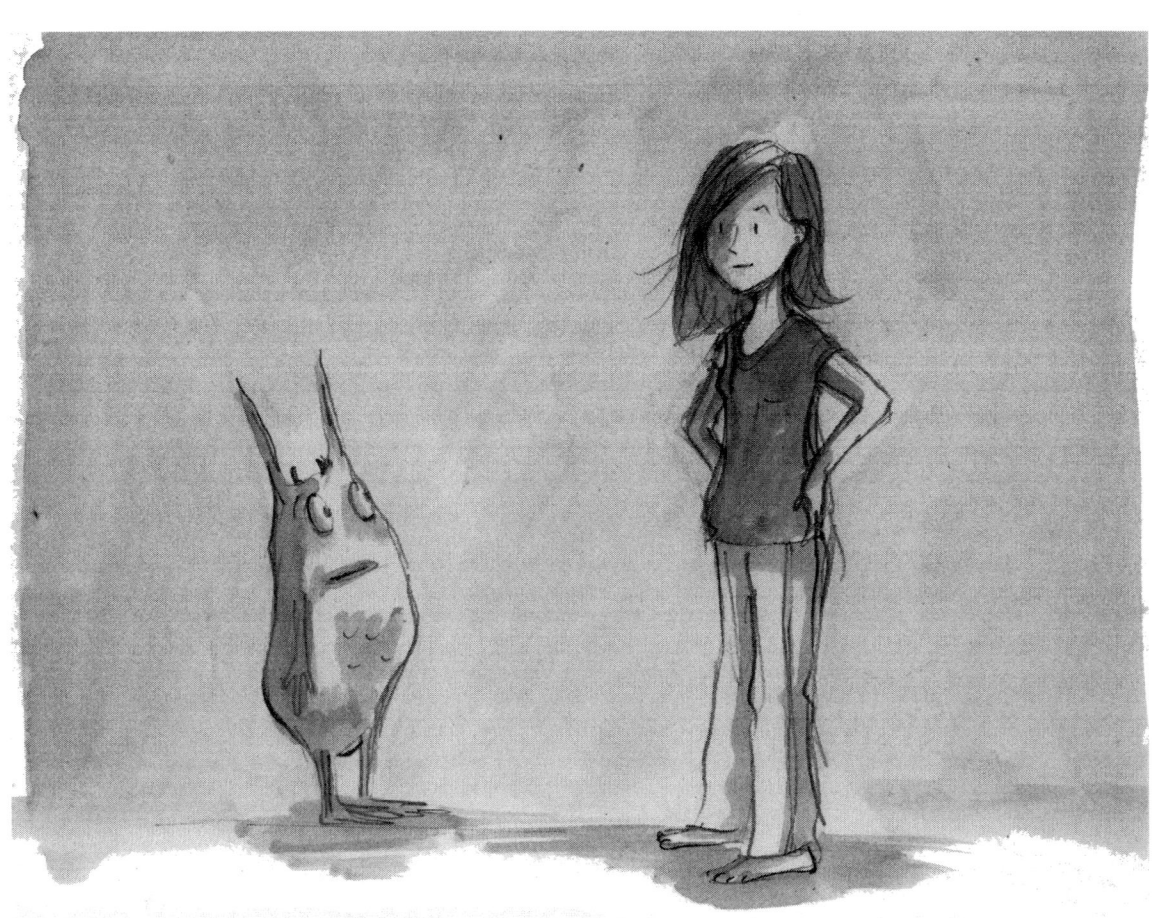

7.1 EPR Activities

i   Everyone should move round the room as if they are monsters (Embodiment) and make loud monster sounds.

ii Use two or more people to create an even bigger monster (Embodiment).

iii Create very large individual or group monsters, using newspaper and masking tape (Projection).

iv Draw, paint or model with clay a very scary monster (Projection).

v   Make use of the movements and models to create a monster story that can be narrated or enacted (Role).

7.2 Worksheet Activities

Use Worksheets 7a to 7i to explore the range of monster-related issues discussed above. For some people the Worksheets provide a more concrete way of working and are specific in their instructions. The Worksheets also suggest possible ways of approaching the topic of overcoming the monster that perhaps have not been considered before.

7a Monsters in the Shadows

7b How I Feel Inside

7c Challenging the Monster

7d Scary Spaces & Places

7e Talking to the Dream Monster

7f The Story of My Monster

7g Scary Shadows

7h Monster Under the Bed

7i Meeting & Welcoming the Monster

Endings: Give everyone the opportunity to write or draw in their notebooks and place any completed worksheets in folders, finish each session with breathing exercises, relaxation under a fleecy blanket, and a calming story (see Section Nine).

Worksheet 7a

Monsters in the Shadows

After a frightening or terrifying experience it often seems that fear exists both on the outside of the person as well as inside the person.

Shadows can be seen in corners and behind curtains, or in a dark street.

We can feel fear in our stomachs or our chests, our hearts may beat faster or we breathe in a panicky way.

Colour or write on the diagram and show where your monsters or shadows live, as well as the spaces that feel OK.

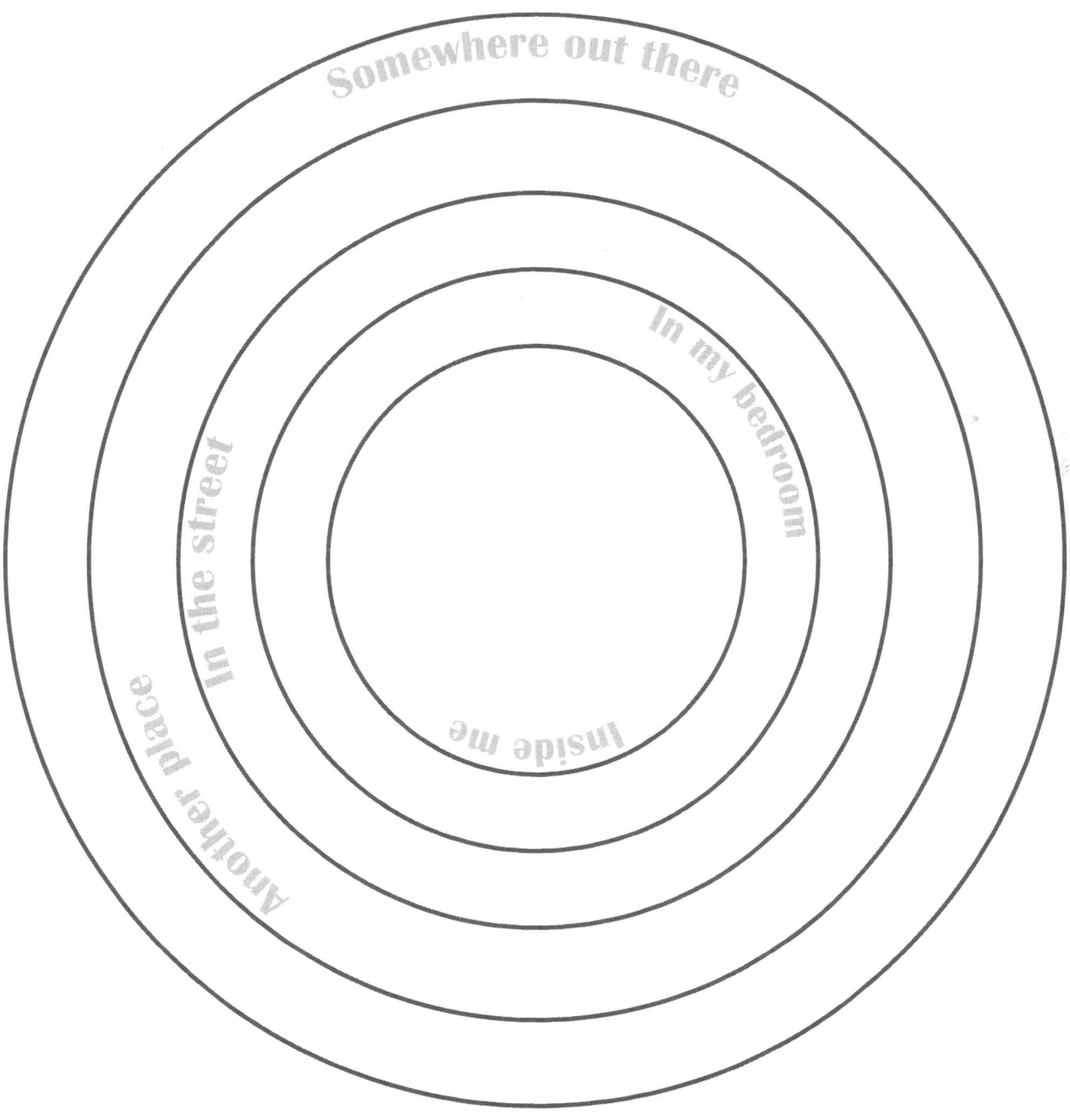

Worksheet 7b
How I Feel Inside

Think about where you feel fear or worries inside you and show them on the picture.

Think about how you feel good inside and show your good feelings on the picture

When you have finished the picture, do some very deep breathing and stretch your body, and then think about this exercise again.

Has anything changed about how you feel inside?

If it has, show the changes on the picture.

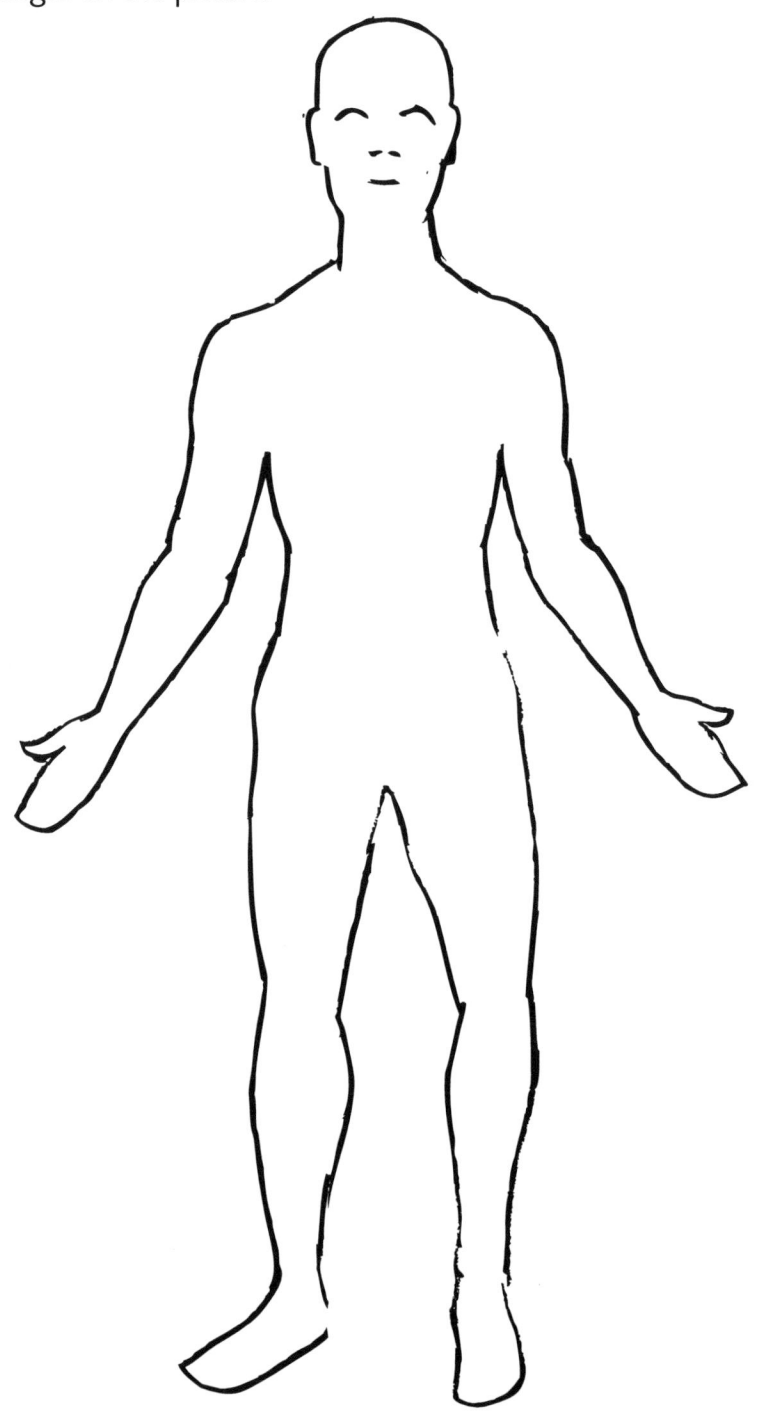

Worksheet 7c
Challenging the Monster

Think about your scary experiences or terrors, making sure you keep your breathing steady. In the circle, create a picture of a monster or alien to represent your terror. Make sure your picture stays inside the circle.

◆ Think about how the monster or alien could change.
◆ Would it be possible to befriend it?
◆ What else could you draw on the picture to help this?

This page may be photocopied for instructional use only. *When the World Falls Apart* © Sue Jennings 2015

Worksheet 7d
Scary Spaces & Places

When you have experienced a terror, sometimes it belongs to a particular place.

Think about your terror and where it belongs: maybe it is something that only happens at school or maybe in the park if you are there alone.

Use the circle below to draw and colour your most scary place.

When you have finished, look at your picture. What must you do to make this space safer and friendlier?

Add something to change the picture to try and make it less scary.

Worksheet 7e

Talking to the Dream Monster

Sometimes if you are having a nightmare, s, you wake up with the feeling of being overpowered or chased or being frozen to the spot with fear.

Try and give a form and shape to your dream monster and draw it in the circle below.

Is it possible to adopt your monster?

Does it have positive qualities?

How could you make your monster more friendly?

(This exercise can be done at home, you could keep a drawing book and pens in your bedroom for when you wake up.)

Worksheet 7f
The Story of My Monster

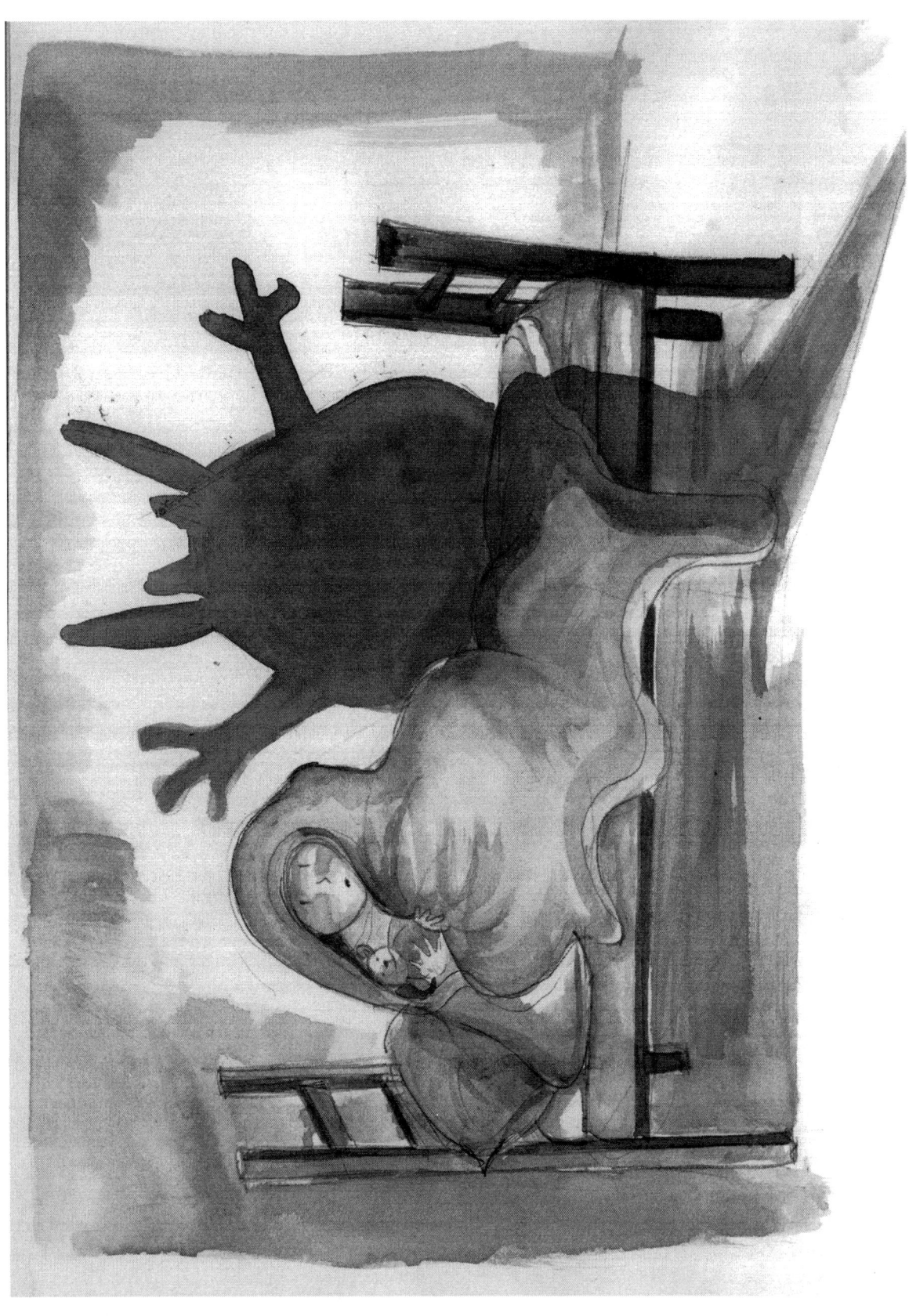

Worksheet 7f

The Story of My Monster

Suitable for Children

Draw a picture of your scary monster and where it lives.

Give your monster a name and write it in big letters.

Draw or write what you want your monster to do.

 This page may be photocopied for instructional use only. *When the World Falls Apart* © Sue Jennings 2015

Worksheet 7g

Scary Shadows

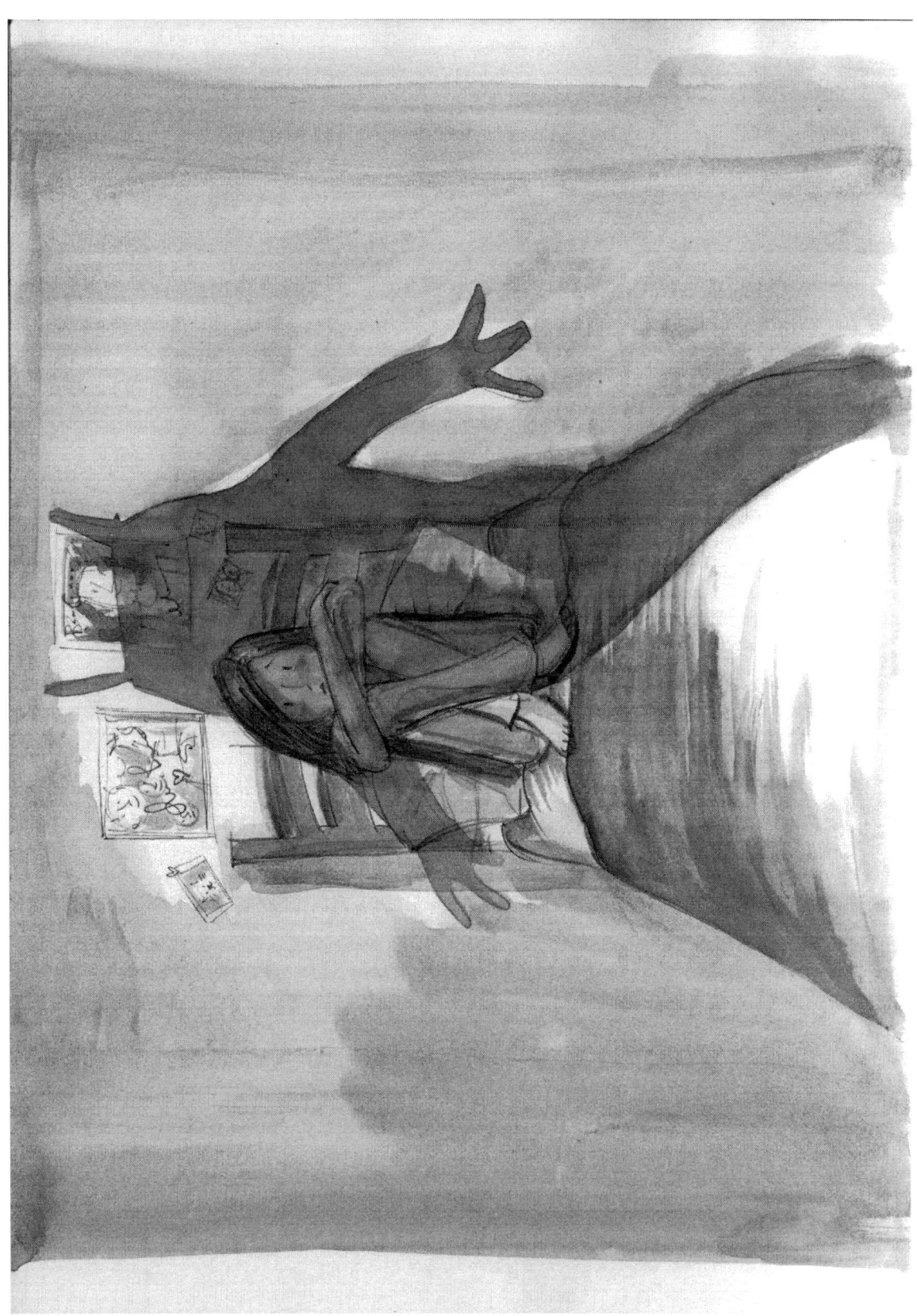

Worksheet 7g
Scary Shadows

Suitable for Teenagers

Draw a picture of your scary shadow and where it lives.

Give your shadow a name and write it in big letters, illustrate your letters if you like.

Draw or write what you want your shadow to do.

Worksheet 7h

Monster Under the Bed

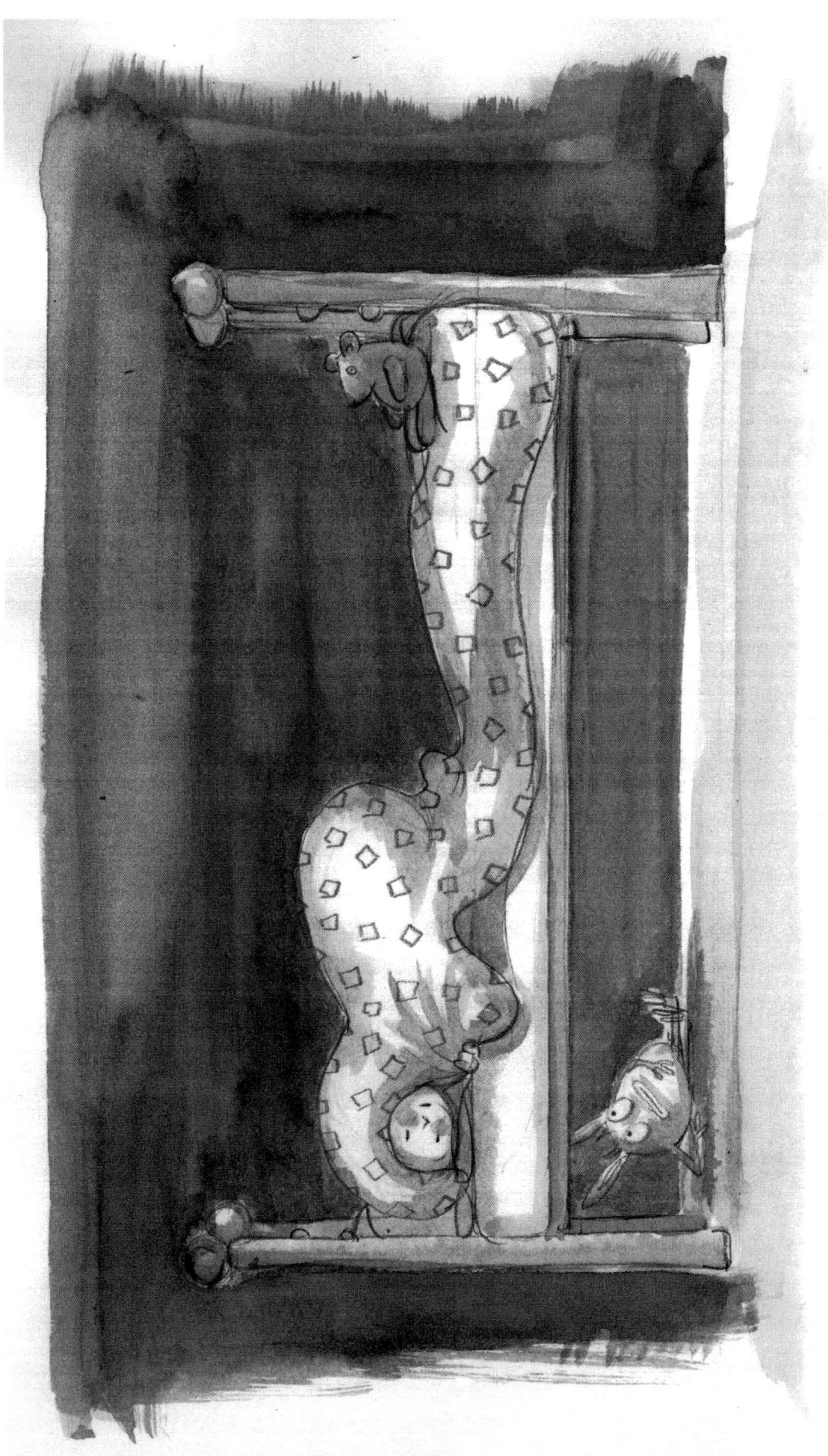

Worksheet 7h

Monster Under the Bed

Suitable for Children

Draw a monster toy that could be your friend.
Maybe you have a cuddly toy that is a bit like a monster.

[ ]

Tell your monster to speak to the monster under the bed and ask why it is there.

Why is the monster there? _____

Maybe the monster has found a place to live that is safe as really he is a scared monster.

Worksheet 7i
Meeting & Welcoming the Monster

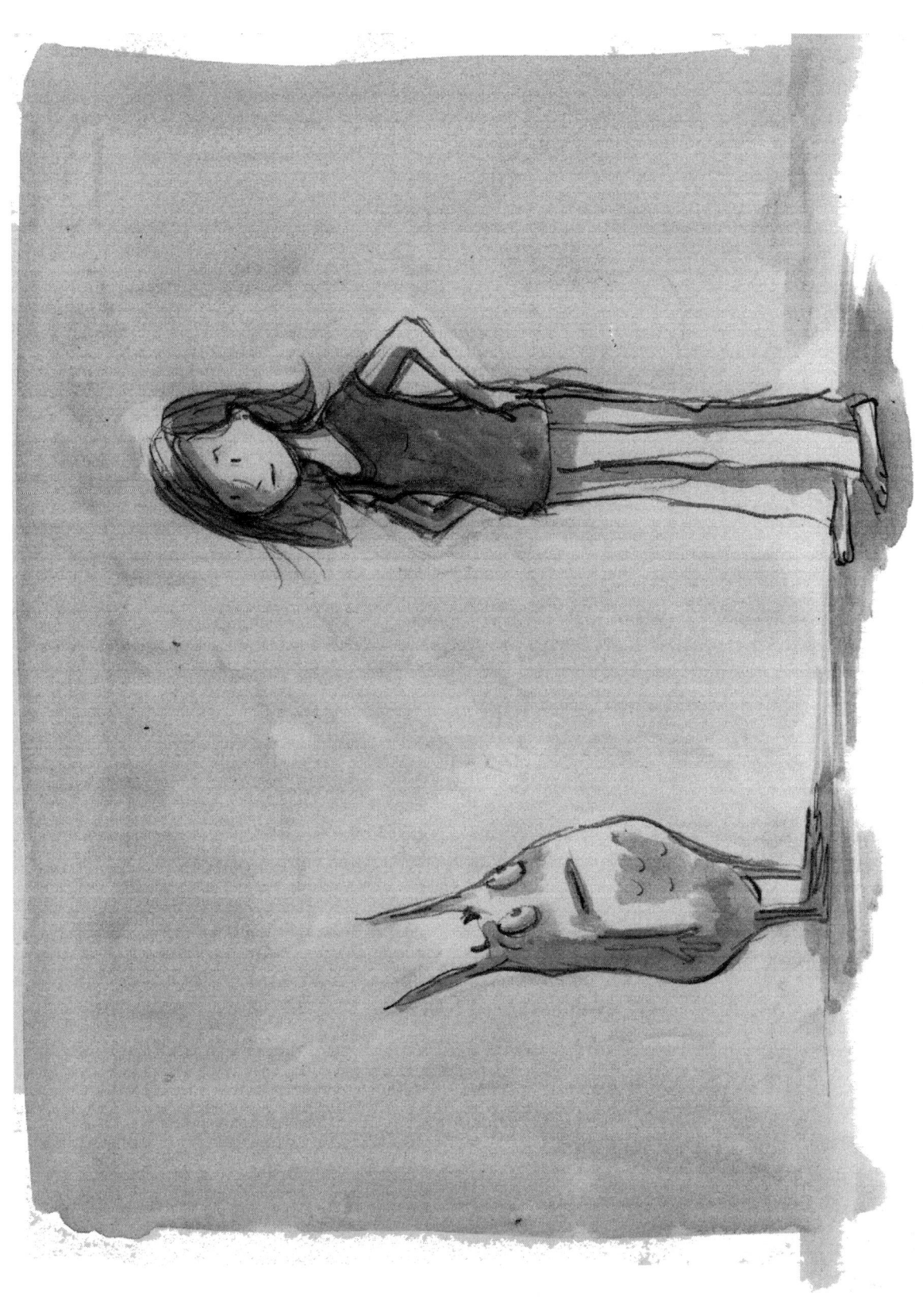

Worksheet 7i

Meeting & Welcoming the Monster

Suitable for Teenagers

Draw a picture of a monster or scary shadow that you are ready to meet.

Breathe deeply and stand up strong in your mind and decide what you will say to this monster or shadow.

Draw or write it here. ─────────────────────────────

Section Eight

Trees

Activities & Worksheets

Activities

8.1 Creating Trees

8.2 Worksheet Activities

Worksheets

8a Falling Leaves

8b Learning to Play

8c Shelters in the Tree

8d Climbing Trees Again

8e Tree of Friends

Section Eight

Trees

Trees are a very helpful symbol to use when considering trauma, as there are many useful examples of trauma being caused by or even to trees. For example, when lightning strikes a tree and the whole tree or a branch falls on someone or their property, or images of trees that have been uprooted by major storms or hurricanes.

However, generally speaking trees are symbols of strength and stability: they have roots that can act as shelters for small creatures; they have strong trunks (as do people), and they have branches that reach out. People talk about the idea of a family tree (although this can be difficult for looked-after children who are severed from their birth tree and do not feel they really belong to the new tree; how does it feel to be grafted on?). Throughout history trees have made good hiding places, and feature in many images and symbols for different countries and cities. A tree is also a relatively simple object to draw, even though people may draw non-naturalistic trees, it does not matter!

Trees

Activities

All of the following exercises are suitable for both Children and Teenagers.

Resources: Worksheets 8a to 8e, for selection where appropriate depending on the experiences of the group, paper, coloured pens, clay or Plasticine, notebooks and folders, soothing music that is not associative. Most CDs of Reiki music are very calming, fleeces, stories from Section Nine Healing Stories.

Ambience: The room needs to be a nurturing space with a range of sensory choices, natural smells such as lavender or rosemary (be sure not to use artificial smells such as air fresheners, and some pot-pourri, as they are a source of many allergies, asthma, and eczema), there needs to be room to move about, with the possibility of snacks such as fresh fruit, and drinks if possible.

Explanation: Discuss with group members how many scary experiences, like the monsters from the previous session, can be transformed when we think about trees. Usually trees are safe place, they can protect us and we can hide inside their trunks or in their branches. Trees are very different from monsters, they are stable and rooted, they protect us, quite the opposite of the monsters!

8.1 Creating Trees

i For children, working in pairs, one person makes the shape of a tree and protects their partner by curling over them.

ii For teenagers, working with a partner, one person stands 'rooted' to the spot and the other tries to dislodge them by gentle pushing (emphasise this is not about chopping down or hacking).

iii Create a picture of a tree that is important to you or to others, by drawing and colouring or modelling: it can be from imaginations or it can really exist.

iv Place all the pictures or models on the floor and each group member can think about and decide where their tree is in relation to the others: whose tree is close to yours and whose is distant?

v Create a story about your tree picture or model and share it with a partner.

8.2 Worksheet Activities

Use Worksheets 8a to 8e to explore some of the security issues discussed above. For some people the Worksheets provide a more concrete way of working and are specific in their instructions. The Worksheets also suggest possible ways of approaching the topic of creating stability that perhaps have not been considered before.

8a Dancing in Circles

8b Learning to Play

8c Shelters in the Tree

8d Climbing Trees Again

8e Tree of Friends

Endings: Give everyone the opportunity to write or draw in their notebook; finish each session with breathing exercises, relaxation under a fleecy blanket, and a calming story (place any Worksheets into folders).

Worksheet 8a
Falling Leaves

The Leaf People have dropped off the tree where they were growing and landed on the ground, there they have found other Leaf People and have started to make friends with everyone. Colour in the picture and think about how this could mirror your own situation.

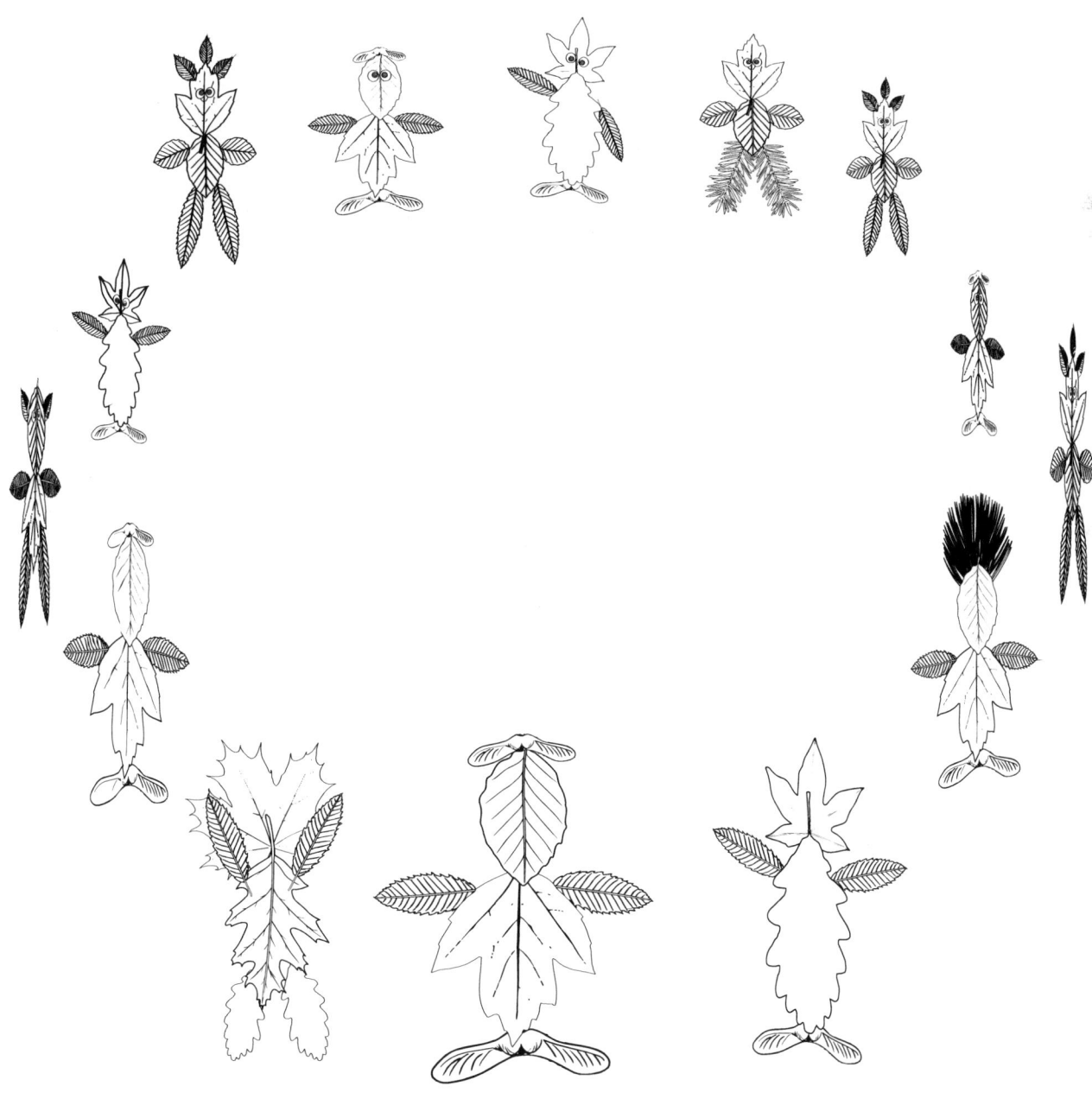

Worksheet 8b
Learning to Play

After scary experiences it is sometimes difficult to play. The Leaf People have been blown off the tree where they were growing and landed on the ground, but they have found each other and started to play.

Colour in the picture and think about the importance of playing.

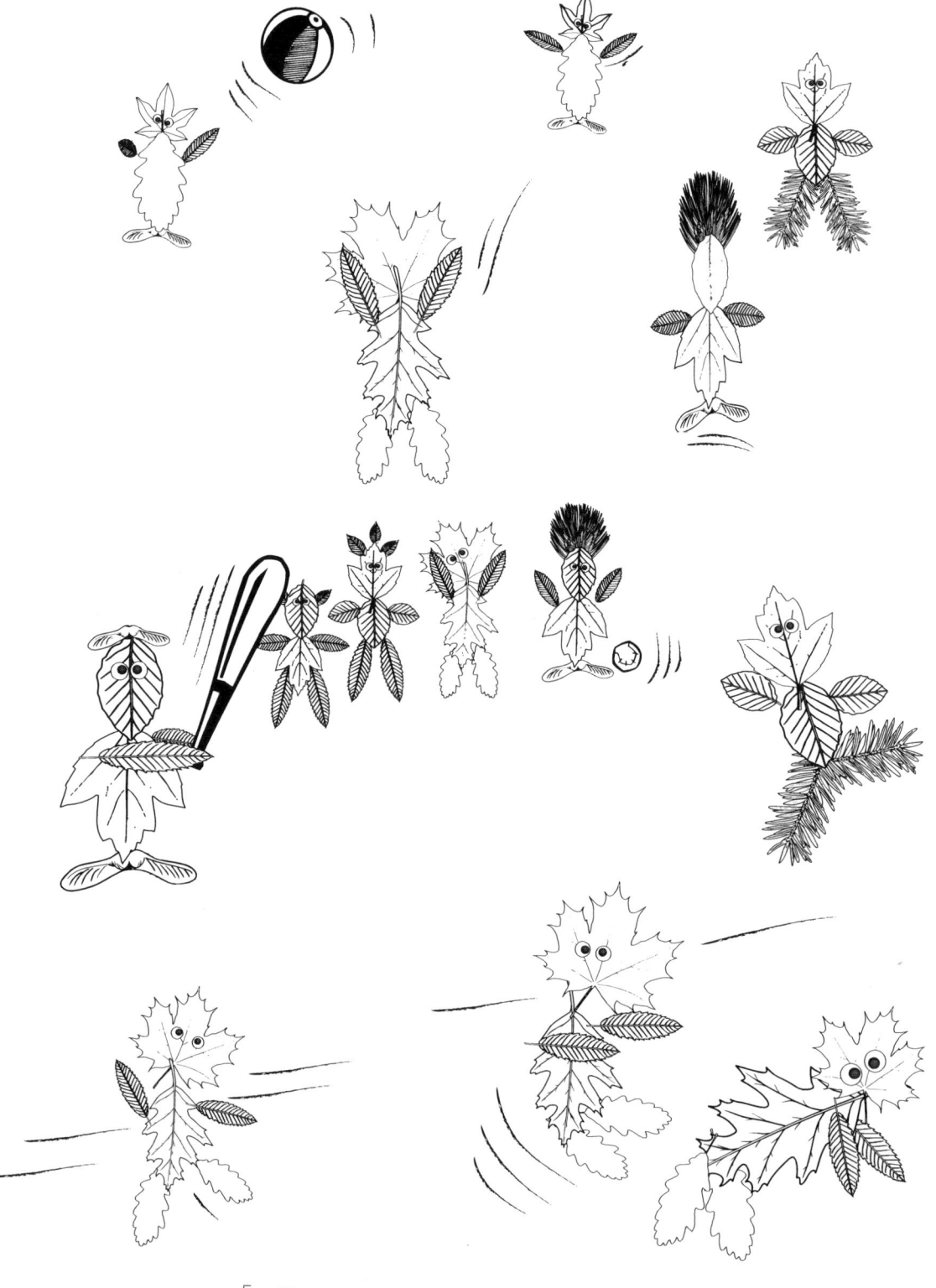

Worksheet 8c
Shelters in the Tree

Often trees can provide safe place to rest or hide, they can offer protection and allow you to see and not be seen.

Look at the tree picture and think where you might build a shelter, somewhere where it is safe to be. It could be in the roots, inside the trunk or in the branches.

Draw your shelter in the tree, you can add anything you like to the picture.

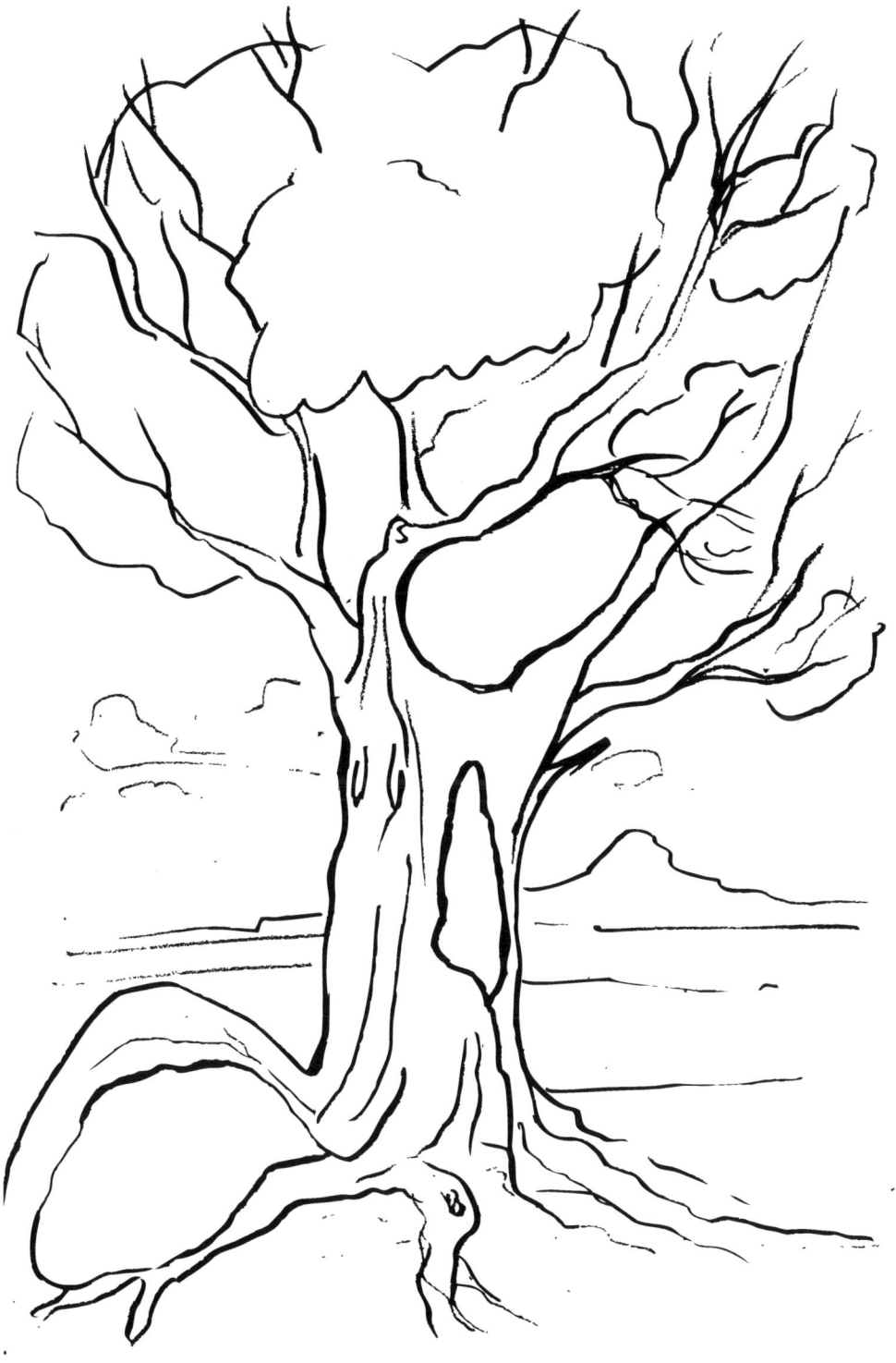

This page may be photocopied for instructional use only. *When the World Falls Apart* © Sue Jennings 2015

Worksheet 8d

Climbing the Tree Again

Think about a tree having deep roots that go far into the ground. Now imagine the strong trunk, and then the branches. The leaves are growing towards the sunshine.

When you have a strong picture in your head, use the trunk below to draw and colour the tree as you imagine it to be.

Where on the tree would you like to be?

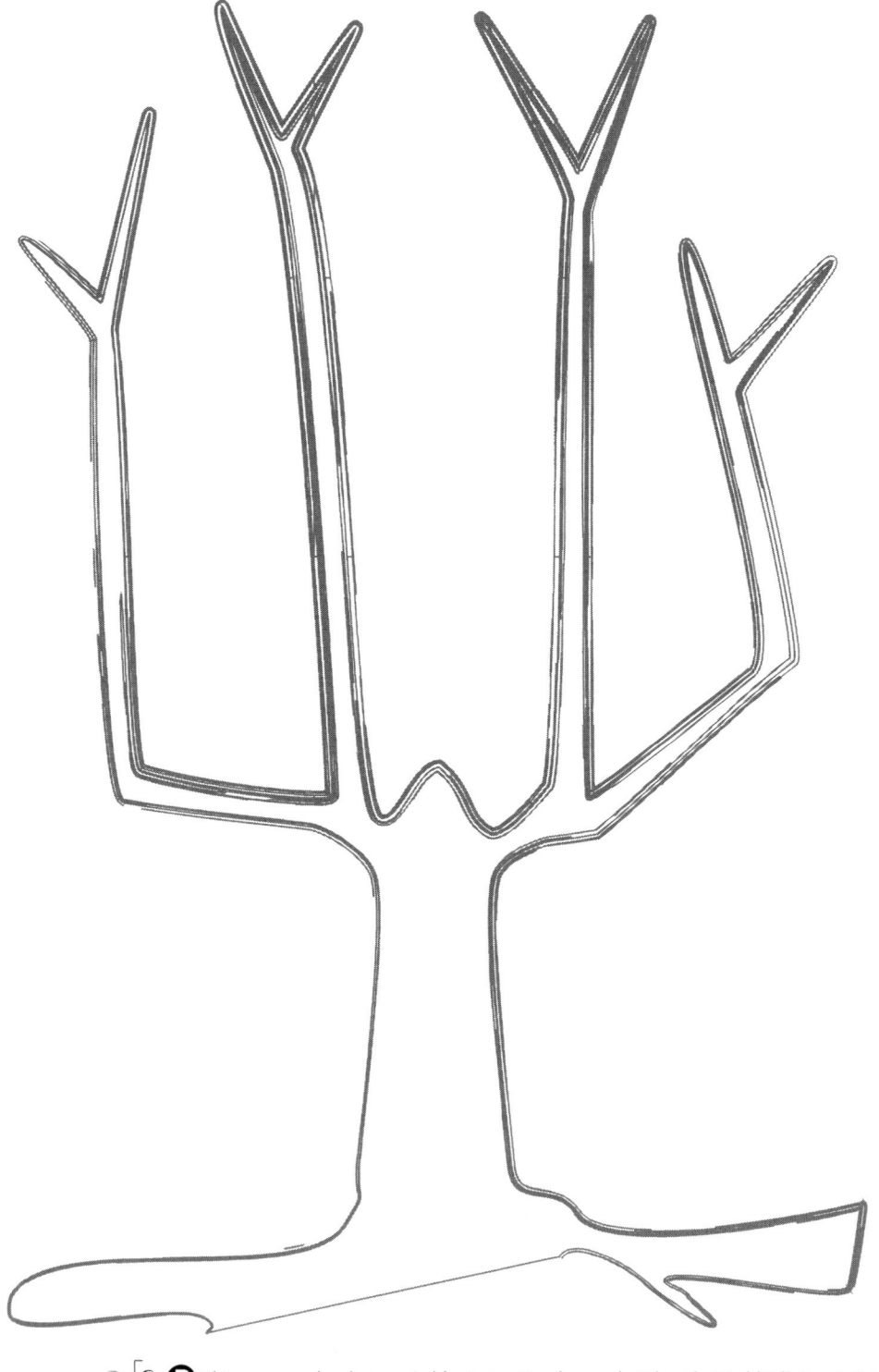

Worksheet 8e
Tree of friends

We are all connected to other people, rather like the branches of a tree. There can be different types of connections that are like trees, for instance there are family trees and friendship trees. Draw or write on the tree to show the special people you are connected to in your life.

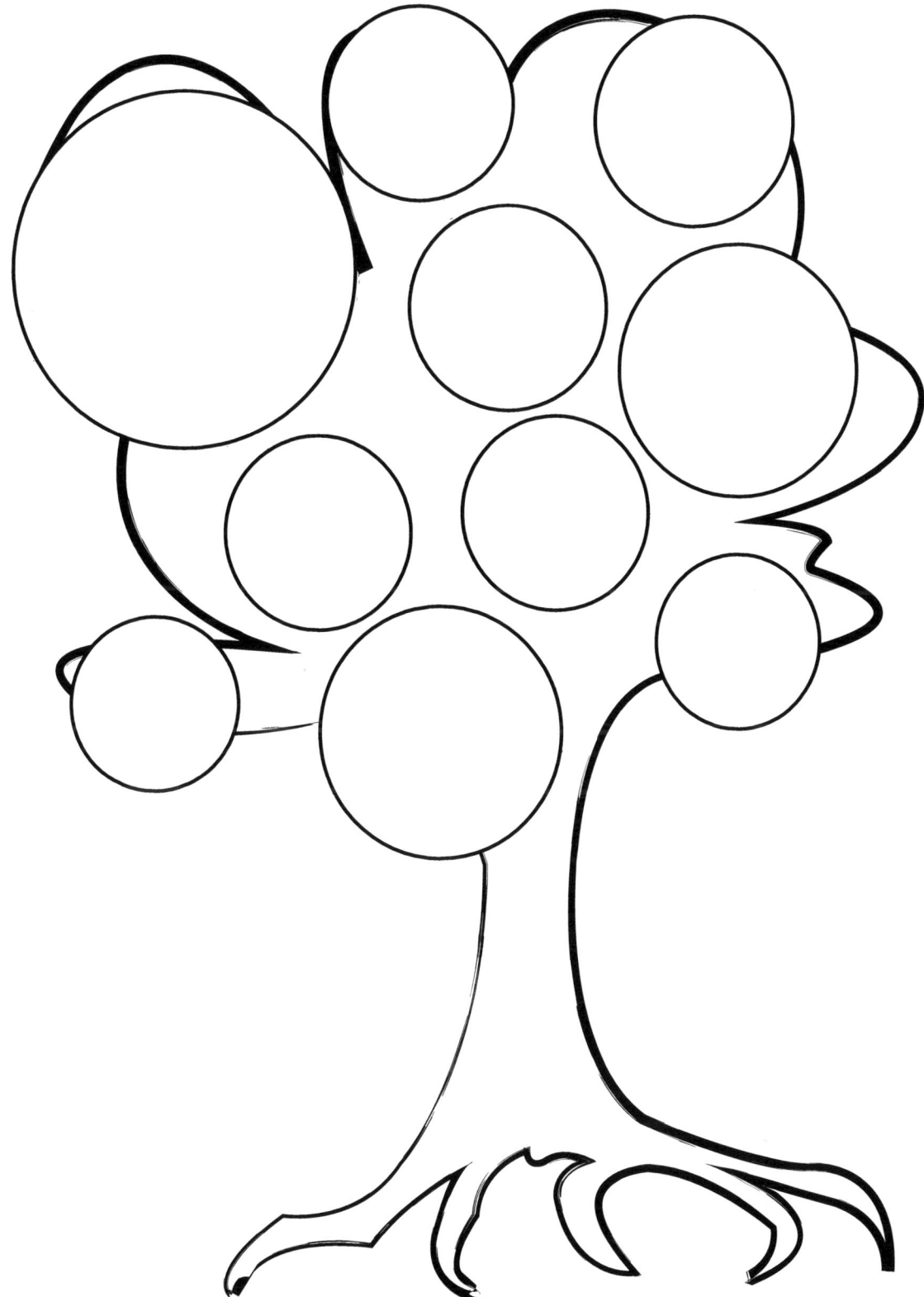

Section Nine

Healing Stories

Stories & Worksheets

Stories

1 The Magic Bag: a Roma Story from Hungary
2 Saint Peter & the Wolves: a traditional story from Romania
3 How Coyote Helped the Karok People to Get Fire: a Native American Story
4 The Flowering Tree: a Tale from South India
5 The Hero's Journey

Worksheets

9a David and Goliath 1
9b David and Goliath 2
9c The Flowering Tree
9d The Story of the Brave Little Goat 1
9e The Story of the Brave Little Goat 2

Section Nine

Healing Stories

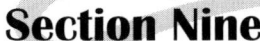

This section focuses on a range of stories from all over the world that can be explored through movement, art and drama, or can be told for their own sake to soothe, for enjoyment or as a 'bedtime story'. Using stories for healing is a very old practice (Jennings 2012) and has been passed down through cultures since ancient times.

It is important to really know your story and also how it can be applied. For example, the story of 'Little Goat' (Worksheet 9d) can be used to build up strengths as well as being suitable as a bedtime story, in contrast, the story of 'The Transformation of Sedna' (Resources, p.133) would need to be used very carefully as there is a major trauma within the story that is eventually transformed. The same consideration should be given to 'The Flowering Tree' (Story 4 and Worksheet 9c), as although it is an excellent story for tackling trauma amongst teenagers, it would not be suitable just as a tale to be told.

Stories can be healing in themselves, but after each story there are themes to explore, and questions that need greater clarification. Always make sure that everyone feels 'grounded' after the telling or exploration of a story.

Many children and young people become very absorbed in a story when it is read to them and need time to 'come out' of their involvement. This process is known as 'grounding' (personal communication with Mary Smail, Director Sesame Institute), whereby participants are able to return to the everyday reality of their surroundings.

One way of doing this is to encourage everyone to focus on sounds they can hear outside the room, then inside the room, and then the sound of their own breathing and heartbeats. They can then stretch and yawn and be invited to discuss or draw the story.

There are several ways of working with the stories and group members can also be encouraged to make their own suggestions. However, initially the story should be read in its entirety by the facilitator, and group members can have their own copy to follow. Some stories may need to be explored over several sessions as they have too many ideas to complete in a single session.

Stories and Worksheets

Resources: Story Sheets 1 to 5 and Worksheets 9a to 9e, for selection where appropriate depending on the experiences of the group, coloured pens, notebooks and folders, soothing music that is not associative. Most CDs of Reiki music are very calming, fleeces.

Ambience: The room needs to be a nurturing space with a range of sensory choices, natural smells such as lavender or rosemary (be sure not to use artificial smells such as air fresheners, and some pot-pourri, as they are a source of many allergies, asthma, and eczema), there needs to be room to move about, with the possibility of snacks such as fresh fruit, and drinks if possible.

Explanation: Discuss with group members how a lot of scary experiences can be like monsters, and that they often occur in stories and are then overcome. Remind people that many story themes are ancient and that even some modern films are based on these ancient tales. Invite people to share stories that they enjoy and see if anyone has a story that really inspires them. Remind them too that they have written stories themselves, and then explain that now it is time to listen to a story from somewhere else.

9.1 Stories

It is helpful to start the practice session with some simple warm-up techniques that are relevant to the story. For example, for the 'The Hero's Journey':

Embodiment techniques

- Imagine you are carrying a heavy rucksack and walk round the room as if the ground is very uneven.
- In pairs, find different ways to cross a fast flowing river.
- Create a scene where you are holding an imaginary rope and your partner is climbing a rock face.

Projective techniques

- Draw a picture of hostile terrain that might be encountered on the journey.
- Create a map for the journey and indicate where there might be difficulties.
- Make a model in clay of the treasure you would like to find at the end of the journey.

Role techniques

- In pairs, one person is a newspaper reporter interviewing the person who has been on the journey.
- In small groups everyone tries to exaggerate in a ridiculous way how difficult the journey was for them.
- In three create a difficult scene on the journey where one person is too scared to go on – what happens?

Every story can have some preparation such as the above, before scenes are created from stories to be explored at greater depth. With 'The Hero's Journey', decide on the stages, write them on the board and then invite small groups to create scenes for each stage. They can be explored in movement or role play.

Page 1 of 2

Story 1 The Magic Bag: a Roma Story from Hungary

This story gives empowerment to marginalised people and empowers them to challenge authority figures. The story can be read as a whole, and then divided into scenes for exploration through movement, drawing and active drama.

Story 2 Saint Peter and the Wolves: a Traditional Story from Romania

This story has a quirky ending and groups can decide what actually happens to Mihai and the old wolf. Group participants usually decide to enlist the intelligence of Mihai and the finer feelings of the old wolf. The story can be read in episodes, and group members can illustrate each episode. Then the whole story can be enacted.

Story 3 How Coyote Helped the Karok People to get Fire: a Native American Story

This is a story about social collaboration, and illustrates how people are able to help each other and can enlist the help of the animals. It is also a trickster story, and shows how tricksters can be clever in the moment to survive. It shows how coyote outwits the hags. It can be enacted by everyone together as the story is being narrated.

Story 4 The Flowering Tree: a Tale from South India

This very powerful story of bullying and cruelty and eventual rescue can be used with teenagers. It needs to be explored over several sessions, taking care that everyone is 'grounded' at the end of each session. This story is important in trauma work as there is healing and recovery at the end. And although there is cruelty, there is also loving support.

Story 5 The Hero's Journey

The stages of the Hero's Journey (Campbell 1993) have been adapted (Schrader 2012) to facilitate personal change and self-learning.

9.2 Worksheets

Use Worksheets 9a to 9e to explore issues that are at the core of traumatic experience. For some people the Worksheets provide a more concrete way of working and are specific in their instructions. The Worksheets also suggest variations on stories and their themes that people may not have considered before.

Usually one story exercise will be sufficient for a single session with discussion and story activities.

9a David and Goliath 1

9b David and Goliath 2

9c The Flowering Tree

9d The Story of the Brave Little Goat 1

9e The Story of the Brave Little Goat 2

Story 1

The Magic Bag: a Roma Story from Hungary

There was once a poor Gipsy family who often went hungry because there was not enough food. Their father worked so hard to look after his family but no matter how hard he worked there was still not enough to care for his wife and children.

One day, he decided to find a solution so he took his axe and went into the forest. He was very angry indeed and his face looked like thunder. There was an old man in the forest with a long white beard who said to the man, 'There is something wrong, please tell me and maybe I could help you'. The father told the old man all about his situation and said just how angry he was that he could not look after his family. The old man went away and came back and handed the father a bag, saying, 'What is inside here will help you – just give it an instruction when you need help'. The father was very grateful and rushed back to show the bag to his family.

His wife looked very disbelieving and said, 'Magic bag – what nonsense – it won't feed the children will it?' The father said to the bag 'Put food on the table for my children – please'. He and his wife could not believe their eyes; wonderful food appeared from the bag until their table was covered. They all sat down and ate a huge meal. And so it went on each day, the bag provided as much food as they could possibly eat.

The man and the woman were sitting down talking one evening and she said 'The King should come and visit us now that life is treating us a bit better'. The man said, 'Why on earth would he want to come to us?' 'Don't forget that he is god-father to our eldest son, of course he will come and visit', she replied. So the next day she put on her best blouse and skirt and walked to the palace.

To begin with, the palace guard would not let her in and said 'What would the King want with the likes of you? Go away and stop bothering me'. 'Please let me through, I have some very important information to tell him and he will be very pleased', she said in a persuasive voice. In the end the guard let her through and she went into the King's chamber in the palace where he was talking with his courtiers and drinking fine wine and eating fine food. She made a low curtsey.

'Hello your Majesty, I have come to bring you to our house. You have not seen your god-son for a long time and he is such a fine boy. We would like to invite you to a meal', she told him. The King really did not want to leave the palace, but in the end he was persuaded and two of the palace guards accompanied him. When they all reached the house and the King entered, the poor man said to the magic bag, 'Provide a meal fit for a king' and immediately the most rich and wonderful food appeared on the table. It was even better food than the King ate at home.

After he had eaten as much as he could the King said to the poor man, 'I want that bag and my guards will take it back to the palace. Thank you for this visit, I have learned a lot'. The family just stood with their mouths open as the King and his guards took the bag and went back home. And sure enough, there was only a small amount of food left and the children soon became hungry. Once again their father took up his axe and went to the forest in a very angry mood.

He met the old man again and told him what had happened, so the old man said to him, 'I will give you another bag but you must look after it and use it wisely. The bag will obey your commands'. The poor man thanked him and started his journey home but he was so curious that he sat down on a bank and looked inside the bag. Immediately two sticks jumped out and began to beat him most cruelly until he was able to say the phrase 'Stop Magic Bag, Stop' to make them stop. He picked up the bag and ran home as fast as he could.

He put the bag on the table and immediately the sticks jumped out and started to beat everyone: mother, father and all the children and they were crying out and shouting, and then he remembered to say 'Stop Magic Bag, Stop'

Then the poor man had an idea and said to his wife 'I am going to the palace; if we don't have food by lunch time then life is a riddle'. He took the bag and went to the palace where he had no trouble getting in to see the King. The King greeted him and said how wonderful the bag was. The man said 'Well, that is just what I am here for. You see I have obtained a much richer bag, very beautiful and lined with silk. Much more fit for a King I think'. The King was very flattered and immediately wanted the new bag lined with silk and he gave the old bag to the poor man. Just as he was leaving the poor man called out, 'Bag do your stuff!' and then he disappeared out of the palace gates.

The sticks jumped out of the bag and began to beat the King and the courtiers and the man could hear everyone squealing and shouting. He ran home as fast as he could and put the bag on the table and asked it to feed his family. There was food on the table once more and the children stopped crying.

The poor man learned a big lesson that day that was, 'Never obey a King who is just being greedy, especially if you are poor yourself'.

Notes

This story gives empowerment to marginalised people and empowers them to challenge authority figures. The story can be read as a whole, and then divided into scenes for exploration through movement, drawing and active drama.

Discussion Points

1. How must it feel to be as hungry as the children are in the story?
2. How must the dad feel that he worked so hard and never earned enough to keep his family?
3. What must it be like to be the King who was so greedy he could not share anything with others?

Exploration

1. Make some hats and crowns that would suit the characters.
2. Draw and colour a poster for the story as a group exercise.
3. Create a drama about the story and take it in turns to play different roles, and express the different emotions.

Story 2

Saint Peter and the Wolves: a traditional story from Romania

It is believed - and why should we argue – that on 16 January, Saint Peter meets with all the wolves in a clearing in the middle of the forest. Wolves come from far and near to hear from Saint Peter about their allocation of food for the year. Maybe it will be a few rabbits or maybe it will be a large red deer or even some sheep from the mountain shepherd. Saint Peter is very wise in the way he shares out the available resources, and the wolves believe that he is always fair. Of course, they always hope that they will have enough food for the year, especially if they have cubs to feed. But they accept his decision.

One year, the day before Saint Peter is due to meet with the wolves, a young shepherd boy called Mihai is feeling rather daring. He wants to know if his father, the chief shepherd, will lose any of his sheep to wolves. Maybe, if he knows in advance, he can find a way to prevent the wolves from taking any sheep and then his father will be very pleased with him.

Mihai slips out from his house early in the morning, before anyone else is awake. All of the sheep are in the large barn. There will be no grass for a few months and then the shepherds will take the sheep up to the mountain meadows and they will stay there for the whole summer. Now though, it is a cold winter and Mihai wraps up warm in his sheepskin cloak.

Mihai travels quickly and quietly through the falling snow and reaches the dense forest. It is drier here and he tries not to slip on the damp beech leaves or trip over new fallen logs. He stops at the clearing to make sure he is alone. No one is in sight, so he swiftly crosses to the other side and climbs up a strong beech tree. He conceals himself on a large branch, against the tree's trunk, making sure he has the whole clearing in view, and waits. He pulls his cloak around him to keep out the bitter cold.

He starts to doze during the long wait but suddenly some new sounds cause him to open his eyes wide. He can hear scuffling and growling, scratching and snapping, and there are dozens of wolves converging on the clearing. And still they come from all sides, some having travelled very long distances. Mihai is amazed at the variety and sizes and ages, and still they come. Everything goes quiet and through the trees, Saint Peter walks towards them. He is wearing his long rough country cloak, and carries his crook made of beech. He stands in the clearing looking firm but kind as the wolves come forward to hear what he will allow them to eat. The list seems endless as Saint Peter gives them roe and red deer, rabbits and rats, sheep and cows, chickens and geese. But no wolf has too many of anything.

Mihai the shepherd boy is getting more and more excited, as none of his father's sheep have been promised to the wolves. Saint Peter is finished now and he is about to leave when a very old wolf appears in the clearing, dragging one of his legs behind him. He says 'I know I am late, but I am old and lame, and the journey has taken me many days; is there anything left for me, or I will surely starve to death'.

Saint Peter looks around him, a little perplexed and then says to the wolf, 'I am afraid there are no more animals to give to the wolves now. Many, many wolves came today from all over the country. Let me see now… Well, all I can tell you is that there is a shepherd boy who is hiding up that tree.'

Notes

This story has a quirky ending and groups can decide what actually happens to Mihai and the old wolf. Group participants usually decide to enlist the intelligence of Mihai and the finer feelings of the old wolf. The story can be read in episodes, and group members can illustrate each episode. Then the whole story can be enacted.

Exploration

1. Invite everyone to create their own ending to the story, suggest that it could be quite unexpected.
2. Sit in a story circle and share the endings.
3. Encourage the group to create a drama from one or more of the endings.

Story 3

How Coyote Helped the Karok People to get Fire: a Native American Story

At the time when there was no fire anywhere on the earth, the people of the Karok tribe suffered greatly. They felt cold and miserable and saw no answer to their situation. Two old hags jealously guarded the fire for it was not to be given to humans. Coyote wanted to help the humans: well, it would keep him in good standing, and he also welcomed opportunities to outwit other creatures. That is the nature of any trickster.

Coyote called a Great Meeting of all the animals to discuss his plan. He placed creatures in a line, from the most strong to the least strong that is, from Lion to Frog, stretching from the Far East to the land of the Karok.

Coyote journeyed to the tepee of the two hags, taking an Indian with him. He concealed the Indian behind the hill and went to the tent and called out 'Good evening: it is bitterly cold out here, would you let me sit by your fire?'

They let him in to lie by the fire as they muttered to themselves, 'He is only a coyote'. He kept watch out of the corner of his eye and tried to plan a means of stealing the fire, and he thought and thought all night. The next day he went to speak with the Indian to make a plan.

As soon as coyote settled in the tepee again, the Indian rushed inside and the two old hags began to pursue him.

Meanwhile Coyote seized a fire stick and rushed away from the Far East. He gave the fire to Lion who went running and gave it to Grizzly Bear who went running and gave it to Cinnamon Bear; he took the fire and went to Wolf, and Wolf took it to Red Squirrel who set his tale alight and forever had a burn mark on his back; Red Squirrel took the fire to Frog who swallowed it in his big mouth; Frog could not run so he jumped. By this time the hags had caught up with them and grabbed Frog by his tail. He jumped again and his tail came away in their hands. Which is why frogs have no tails to this very day.

Frog kept the fire safe inside him while he swam underwater until it was safe. He spat the fire into a pile of dry brushwood and there it rests to this day.

There is always fire inside dry wood and to make it come out, the Indians rub two sticks together to light their fires.

Notes

This is a story about social collaboration, and illustrates how people are able to help each other and can enlist the help of the animals. It is also a trickster story, and shows how tricksters can be clever in the moment to survive. It shows how coyote outwits the hags. It can be enacted by everyone together as the story is being narrated.

Discussion

1. What must it feel like when the hags say 'He's only a coyote'?
2. Are the animals really able to collaborate?
3. What might happen to the hags?

Exploration

1. Explore the story through movement for each of the animals, making them larger than life.
2. Using card, pens and string, create masks of the animals.
3. Make a play using the movement, the masks and the story.

Story 4

The Flowering Tree: a Tale from South India

This story can also be used in conjunction with Worksheet 9c. It is a story that illustrates bullying amongst girls of a similar age, and how an individual can lose all sense of self when they are undermined and intimidated, especially through jealousy.

In ancient times there lived a king and his two daughters and son. The eldest daughter was married and lived in another town. There was also a poor woman who had two daughters and slaved night and day to keep them fed and clothed.

One day, the poor woman's younger daughter said to her sister, 'I know a way that we can help our mother: I will turn into a flowering tree and you can pick all the flowers and sell them'. She instructed her sister to fetch two jars of water, making sure the water was not touched by hand, and the younger sister meditated and chanted.

'Pour the contents of the first jar over me, and then pick all the flowers very carefully without damaging my leaves or branches; then pour the second one and I will become myself again'. The older sister did just that and was amazed that her younger sister turned into a most beautiful tree, all covered in blossoms.

'You see how easy it is? Now take the flowers and you will see that people will want to buy them'. So the older sister took the flowers to the palace, calling out that she had flowers for sale. The Queen and her younger daughter looked out and sent a servant to purchase them. The sisters decided to hide the money while they continued to create and sell the flowers. Soon they had five fistfuls of coins, as each day the younger sister turned into the flowering tree and then back again.

The Prince began to notice the young flower seller and was very curious; one day he followed her back to her dwelling and was surprised to find that there were no flowering trees to be seen. He concealed himself in the large tree in the garden and watched and waited. The next day he was most surprised to see the young girl sit under the tree while her sister poured the water over her, picked her blossoms and then poured the second jar, and he later let his father know that he would be married.

The King sent for the mother of the two sisters and asked her the truth of what his son was saying. Their mother of course knew nothing about it, and went home very angry. She called her daughters and asked them, so the two sisters showed their mother the truth and gave her the money.

The younger sister and the Prince were married in a wonderful ceremony, and that night they both lay on their bed without a word to say to each other. After several nights, the younger sister broke the silence, 'What shall we say to each other?' The Prince said, 'I want you to turn into the flowering tree'. He said they could cover their bed with beautiful flowers; so she agreed and explained to him how to take care of her leaves and branches.

Each morning they shook the old flowers out of the window, and picked fresh flowers each night. The wilting flowers were noticed by the Prince's younger sister who was already jealous, and she spied through the door. She was determined to take her sister-in-law to meet her friends in the park.

The other girls were playing together amongst the trees. 'Come and meet my sister-in-law – she knows how to turn into a tree. You can all get flowers for your hair. I have seen you change into a flowering tree', taunted the younger Princess. 'You have to do it, we will fetch the water pots'. The girls carelessly tipped the water over her and grabbed the flowers, breaking leaves and branches. They were laughing and pushing each other as they stripped the tree bare. Then they threw the second pot of water over her and ran back to the palace.

She slowly and painfully turned back into herself again, but she was very damaged: she had no hands or feet and could only moan and sigh, yet her face was as beautiful as ever. She had become a Thing and no longer a special young woman. A kindly gardener found her and picked her up and carried her to the edge of the road, saying 'Someone will find you soon and care for you'.

The younger Princess went back to the palace, and when her mother asked where her daughter-in-law was the girl said carelessly, 'Oh, we all came back on our own – I don't know where she is'. Her brother, the Prince, asked the same question when he returned home that night. The Prince was distraught and took the robes of an ascetic and went walking from place to place to look for his wife for he truly loved her.

Meanwhile the Thing lay at the road side, moaning pitifully. After some hours a farmer came along with his horse and cart. He noticed the Thing lying at the roadside and felt sorry for her. He picked her up very tenderly and placed her in his cart. He was travelling to the next town and decided to place her at the palace gates where surely someone would look after her. The servants from the palace noticed her and told their Queen, suggesting they should bring her inside. Initially the Queen refused but finally was persuaded, providing the servants took good care of her. But when the Queen saw her face, she was sure that the Thing was her brother's wife. She was indeed the older married sister of the Prince and lived in another town. They cared for the Thing as best they could while the Queen pondered what she should do.

The Prince was still wandering the roads looking for his wife and living in discomfort as a poor man. Finally, he came to the town where his older sister lived and went to beg at the palace and inquire after his wife. The Queen welcomed him into the house and said that there was someone he should see. She led him to the room where the Thing was lying on a bed, her wrists and ankles slowly healing with the tender care of the servants. The Prince recognised his wife immediately and swept her up in his arms, 'Tell me what I must do!' he said, once they were alone.

Her voice came back and she said that he must do exactly as he had done before but take even more care with the pouring of the water as she was in much pain. She meditated while he fetched two jars and tenderly poured the water over her. Slowly she turned into the flowering tree again and all her leaves and branches grew intact. He did not pick any flowers but just as gently poured the second jar of water. She returned to herself again, with hands and feet and not a scar in sight.

They were joyfully reunited together and returned to their own town having celebrated with the Prince's older sister, and rewarding the servants for their care. When the King heard what had happened he was furious and banished his youngest daughter outside the walls of the town. In time, the Prince became King and ruled wisely and justly with his flowering wife at his side.

Notes

This very powerful story of bullying and cruelty and eventual rescue can be used with teenagers. It needs to be explored over several sessions, taking care that everyone is 'grounded' at the end of each session. This story is important in trauma work as there is healing and recovery at the end. And although there is cruelty, there is also loving support.

Exploration

1. This is a very sensory story and group members can prepare by having some sensory play with different textures.
2. A narrator can tell the story while it is being expressed non-verbally by the group.
3. Paint a group picture that integrates all aspects of the story.
4. In pairs, participants can discuss different scenes: the reaction of the mother when she discovers what her daughters have been doing, (despite the fact they were trying to be helpful); the conversation between the younger sister and her friends when she is planning to be cruel to the flowering girl (including her feelings of being jealous of her brother getting married).
5. Dramatise the story with small groups of participants.
6. Tell the story from the point of view of a young servant-girl who lives in the palace.

Story 5

The Hero's Journey

The stages of the Hero's Journey (Campbell 1993) have been adapted (Schrader 2012) to facilitate personal change and self-learning. The number of stages of the journey can vary from 6 to 11, but the following key points provide the basic structure. These stages are illustrated in many myths and stories when the hero or heroine embarks on a quest to find treasure, encounters and overcomes danger, and then returns home with new learning. The stages can be explored through any art activities : dance, movement, play, painting, drama, storytelling, or a combination of them all. There is an elaborated Hero's Journey in *101 Ideas for Managing Challenging Behaviour* (Jennings 2013). You can use the following key points to construct a story:

1 Call to go on the journey, and preparation.
2 The difficult road and encounter with danger.
3 Call for help to overcome the danger.
4 Discovering the treasure.
5 Returning home to share the story.

It is very important for participants to write in their notebooks during the journey, rather like creating a log of their journey. After completing this sort of exercise people often find that they have been able to move beyond the trauma and find a new way of being. Sometimes the trauma itself is the danger in the journey, perceived as a dragon or mythic monster. A call for help enables the individual to find support to overcome the danger. The treasure that is found is often the treasure within each and every one of us, and we are able to return feeling valued and confident with a story to tell. Stage 5 is writing the story of the whole journey and sharing it with a partner. Another way is to create a drama of the journey with a small group and share it with the whole group.

Worksheet 9a
David and Goliath 1

In this story from the Bible, a huge giant called Goliath is facing an army who are afraid to fight him. A boy called David accepts the challenge to fight the giant, armed only with a slingshot. Colour the giant and David and remember how David was very clever in finding a way to overcome the giant.

Colour the two people in your choice of colours.

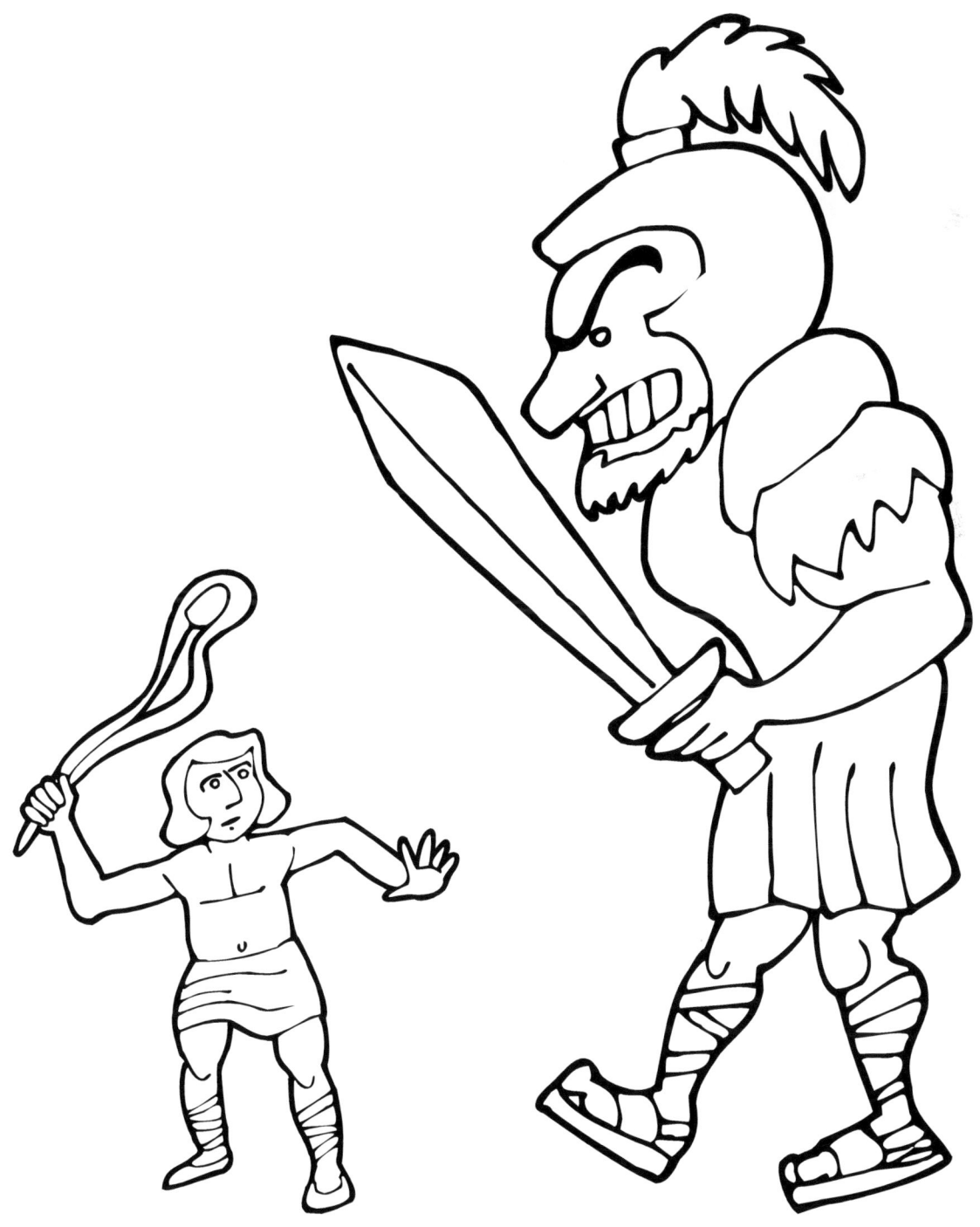

Worksheet 9b
David and Goliath 2

How do you think David was feeling when he overcame the giant with such a simple idea? Sometimes when our fears seem huge we can think of a simple solution like David's.

Colour David to show he has overcome the giant, and colour Goliath to show he has failed!

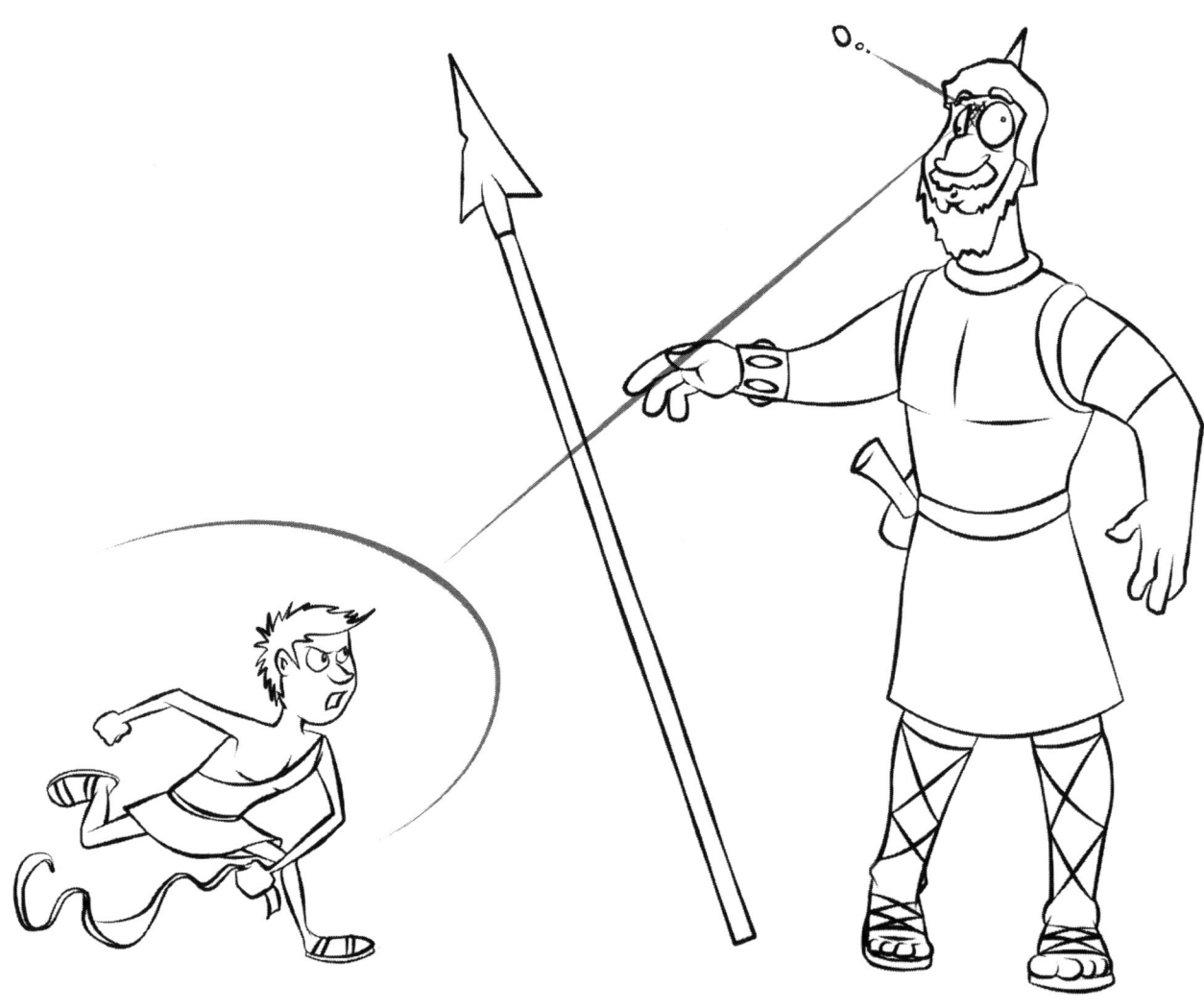

Worksheet 9c

The Flowering Tree

This story is about being bullied by teenagers like ourselves.
It shows how someone eventually overcame the bullies and survived, and how it was important that she was loved and cared for by both strangers and friends.

Colour the tree to show the most beautiful flowers you can think of.

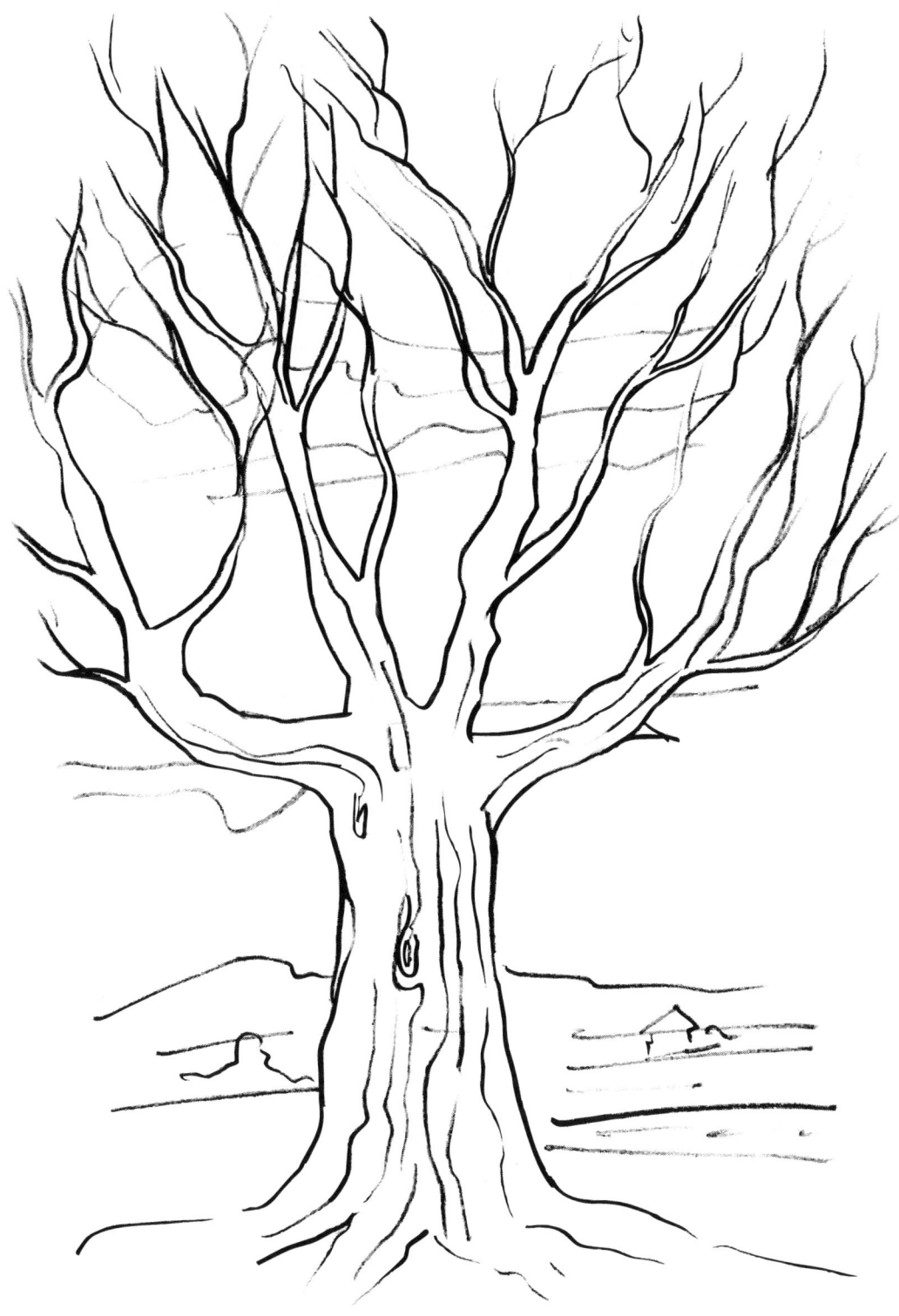

Worksheet 9d

The Story of the Brave Little Goat 1

The Little Goat was the smallest of the flock but he was very brave. He was also very clever and he saved the other goats from being eaten by the farmer as well as from the scary tiger. He could always think ahead and then think of a plan that would trick the other creatures who could be dangerous.

Colour the picture which is a scene from the story

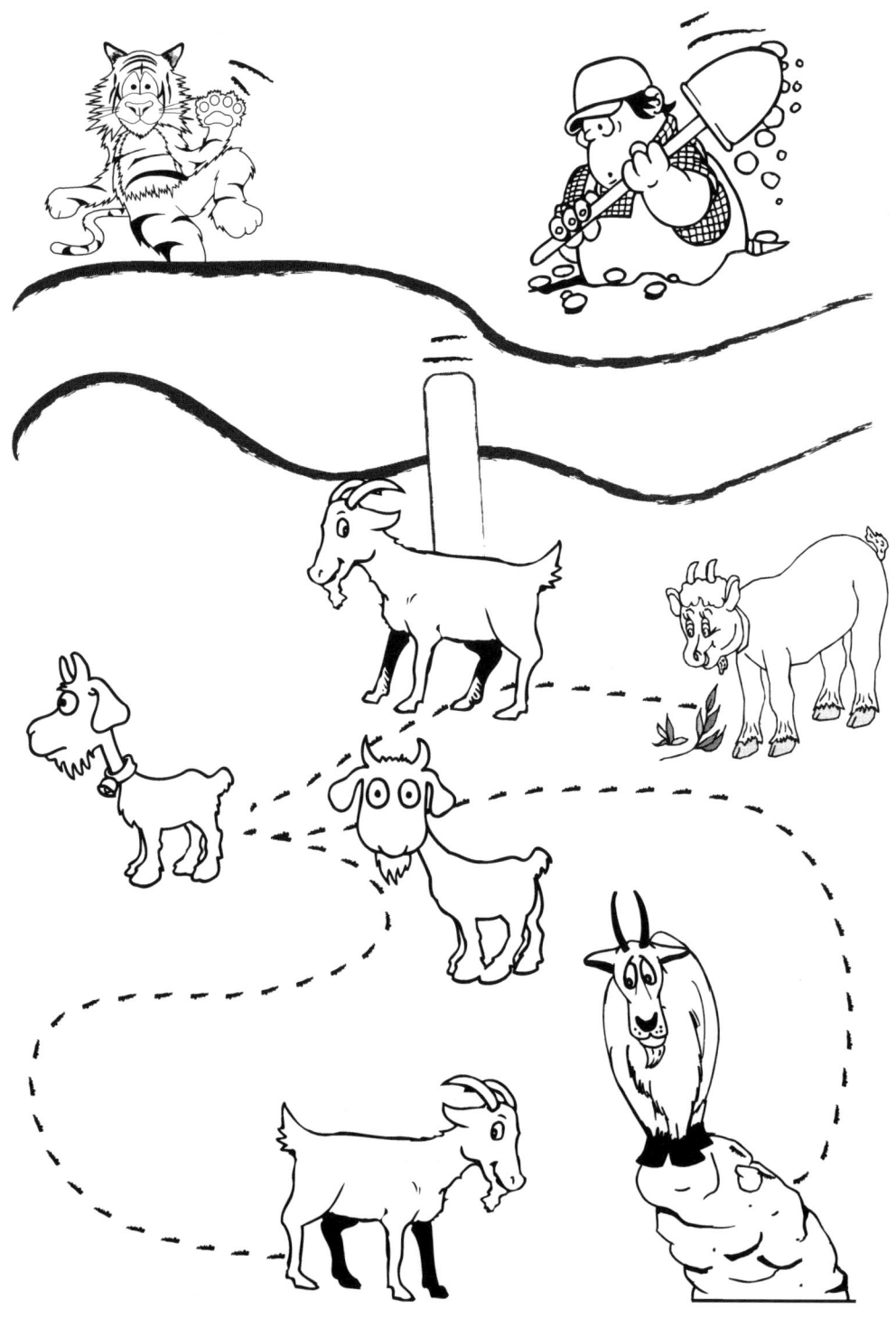

Worksheet 9e

The Story of the Brave Little Goat 2

After Little Goat had brought all the goats to safety, away from the farm, they lived in a field near the river. Little Goat knew that tiger was watching them, even though he was hiding in the tall grass at the edge of the river.

This is another pictures from the story to colour

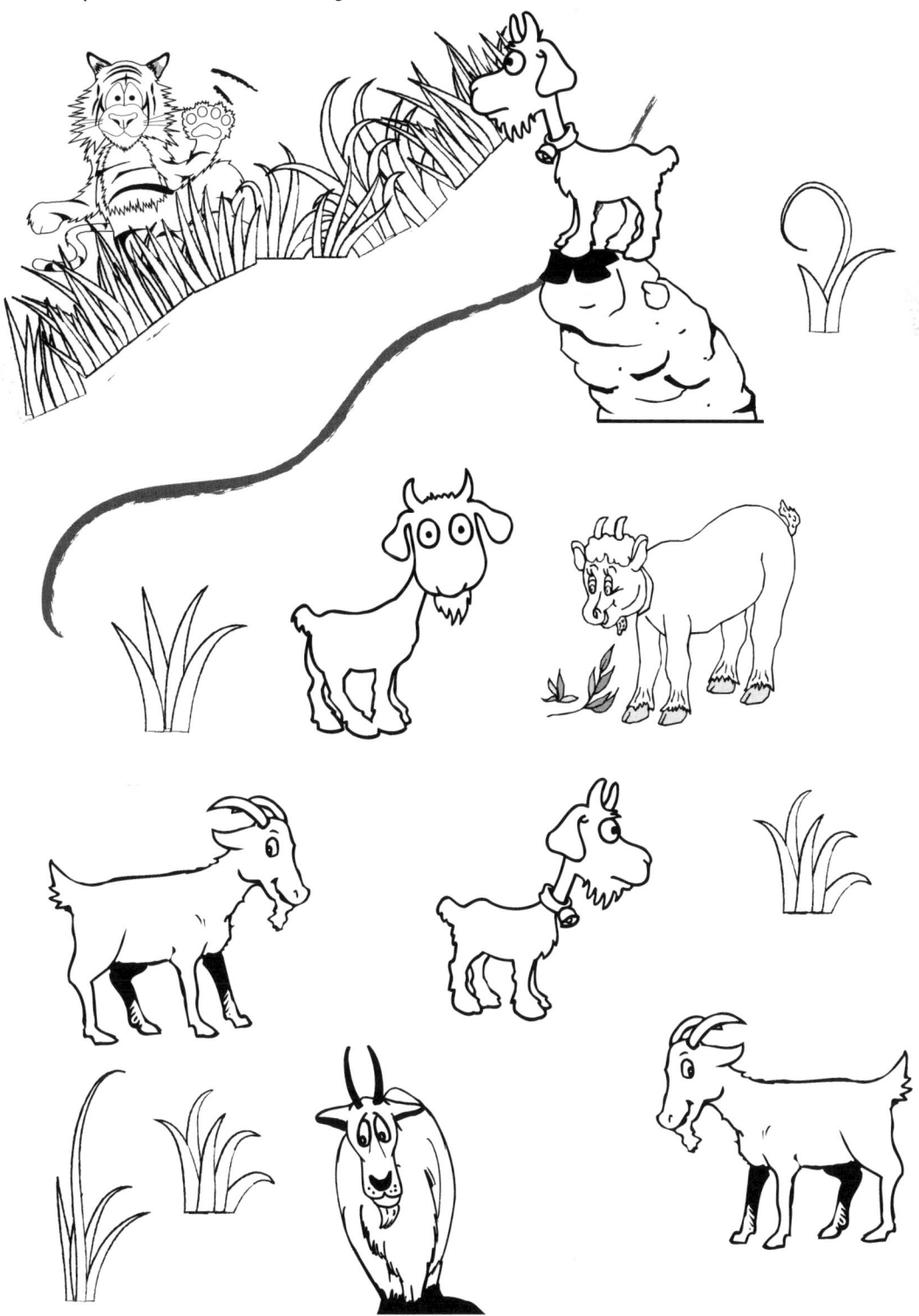

Resources

Group Contract & Agreement

We are attending the group on the following dates:
_____

We all agree to abide by the group rules as follows:

1. Everyone listens to what other people are saying without interrupting

2. Everyone agrees to behave in a respectful manner to others

3. Everyone agrees that there is no verbal or physical violence

4. Everyone agrees that equipment is not to be broken

5. _____

6. _____

7. _____

8. _____

9. _____

Signature or Thumb Print from all Group Members:

Additional Healing Story 1

The Transformation of Sedna (an Inuit story)

Suitable for Older Teenagers

This story contains severe trauma and needs to be used with care. However, the transformation enables young people to experience that change is possible after trauma.

Sedna, a beautiful young woman, is thinking that it is time to leave home and marry and settle down. None of the young men who come to visit her pleases her until one day she spies a handsome stranger in the distance. She agrees to go to his home and he removes his cloak and puts it round her shoulders. He then changes into the stormy petrel bird and flies with her to his nest on the cliff tops. The nest is very dirty and Sedna wishes that she had never come, and she sends a message out through the air and hopes that her father can hear it.

Her father does hear her and takes his kayak and rows to where she is waiting nervously, as the petrel is only out of the nest for a short time. She clambers down into the boat and her father starts to row. The bird sees them and dives down closely because he loves Sedna very much. There is a storm blowing up and her father becomes scared and wishes he had never come. He pushes her out of the boat hoping it will appease both the bird and the storm. Sedna hangs on with her fingers clasped around the edge of the boat but her father will have none of it. He takes out his axe and with a swift blow he cuts off her fingers. Sedna holds on again with her other hand and her father hits again and then again. Three times and all her fingers have gone to the bottom of the sea and turned into sea creatures.

Sedna herself floats to the seabed and she gradually turns into a mermaid or silkie and befriends all the animals under the sea who in time love her dearly. She looks after the land and land-animals, and the hunters have to ask her permission to hunt. If they break the traditional rules of hunting, Sedna will send terrible storms and the local shaman has to visit her to intercede on their behalf.

The shaman has to journey through many difficulties to meet her, including a overcoming a scalding cauldron and a fierce dog. His first task is to comb all the seaweed out of her hair because she has no hands. Then and only then will she listen to his request.

In the end, Sedna forgives her father for the terrible deed of chopping off all her fingers but she stays with the myriad of sea-creatures, who are, after all, a part of her. She continues to punish hunters who neglect to care for nature and she tells wonderful stories to her sea friends.

Page 1 of 2

Notes

There are many themes in this story including the power of men over women, (both Sedna's father and the stormy petrel) while she is still a teenager; empowerment of women as Sedna learns to nurture herself and also care for the sea-creatures; Sedna takes charge of the care of the environment and is the negotiator with the shaman; she also allows him to care for her.

Exploration

There are several scenes in this story that can be made into a dramatic scene and enacted. One group used five people to all create together the person of Sedna, (three created her hair). The enactment can use words or mime or movement.

i   This story is very physical and can be acted out and 'moved' through each scene.
ii Working in pairs, enact the scene where the shaman has to comb the sea-weed out of Sedna's hair.
iii Create a group picture of Sedna as a collaborative endeavour (using paint, collage materials).
iv Scenes from the story can be enacted through 'body-sculpts' or movement.
v   The whole story can be enacted with a series of scenes. (Large pieces of soft material would be useful for the enactments e.g., blue or green for creating waves and storms.)

Feedback from a participant

On first hearing the story of Sedna, I was shocked to hear how her own father had chopped off her fingers to save himself from the stormy petrel instead of saving his own daughter. I was very sad to realise how this affected even being unable to comb her own hair. The transformation to mermaid and her survival was heartening as was her new vocation to look after the small sea creatures.

From a personal perspective, I can identify with Sedna as it was my own father who betrayed me with abuse instead of trustworthiness. My life became transformed into survival. My relationships and sexuality were affected and my marriage was failing. Suicide was a real temptation at one point. Eventually, like Sedna, I had help and allowed others to assist me, just as Sedna had allowed the shaman to comb her hair. Now although I still have difficulty forgiving my father (now dead), I do not feel angry or vengeful towards him or project this on to others. I enjoy my relationships, and as Sedna looked after the vulnerable creatures, my work is to care for my family and help troubled children.

I found using the story very moving and empowering as I realise how far I have come on my own journey and formed bonds with others in the groups.

Additional Healing Story 2

The Story of the Brave Little Goat

Why the Tapir has no Tail (a Malay story)

On the goat farm was a large herd of goats, who were well fed and content. One goat, known as Thin Goat, would keep alert and know what was going on. He was called Thin Goat because no matter what he ate, he never grew any fatter! One night he heard the farmer and his wife talking, they were planning a dinner party and he was going to be the meat. Quickly, he woke the other goats and called them to a meeting: 'Listen,' he said, 'I have just heard the farmer planning to kill and eat me for supper – even if I escape, then he will start to eat you instead.' All the goats looked shocked and scared and were speechless. Thin Goat continued, 'I have a plan but you must all be very, very quiet. At midnight I will force open the gate and we will all escape to a new land, without making a sound. Trust me.'

They did just that and without making a sound, Thin Goat forced open the gate, all of the herd followed him and they started to run as fast as they could. Eventually, and with great tiredness they came to a large green and grassy field with a lake nearby. Thin Goat said, 'This will make us a perfect home.' All the goats relaxed, and ate the luscious green grass and drank from the lake.

Thin Goat was ever watchful and noticed some movement at the edge of the field and he knew it was Tiger, and tigers are very dangerous to goats: they also like to eat them for dinner. Thin Goat started to speak in a very loud voice and hoped the other goats would follow him: 'Hello Mr Tiger! I would not wait there if I were you, we goats are very, very hungry and are all ready to charge you and trample you down.' The other goats realised what Thin Goat was doing and shouted out VERY, VERY, LOUDLY! 'Right goats, let's charge the tiger so we can eat him for dinner.' The Tiger could not believe what he was hearing – goats eating tigers – surely it was the other way round, 'Eek!' Here they were charging towards him, shouting and their hoofs making a terrible noise on the ground. He turned and fled, terrified he would be killed by goats. He went into the forest and kept running until he could run no more.

He paused for breath, but looked fearfully around him. A Tapir came towards him and asked what on earth was going on, and Tiger explained about the goats. Tapir laughed and laughed, 'What nonsense he said, goats cannot kill tigers, let alone eat them!' 'You have not seen them,' said Tiger, 'You would know that I was right if you saw them.' 'All right,' said Tapir, 'We will go together and you will show me and I will show you there is nothing to be afraid of, goats eating tigers indeed!'

Tiger agreed to go back with Tapir, but only if Tapir agreed they could tie their tails together, so Tapir would have to look after him. He wasn't going to take any risks! They journeyed back to the field which took a little while as they managed their tied tails! Meanwhile, Thin Goat was keeping guard on a nearby hill as he expected Tiger to return. Sure enough, he spied Tiger and Tapir, so he called to the goats, 'Go to the edge of the forest and eat as many red berries as you, really scrunch and munch them.' The goats did just that, really enjoying the fruits, and as the Tiger and Tapir got close, Thin Goat said quietly, 'Quickly, all run together towards the forest'.

He called out in his loud voice, 'Hello Mr Tiger, we have just eaten your grandfather, and now I think we will start on you and your friend Tapir'. Tiger and Tapir looked aghast, thinking that blood was dripping from the goats' mouths and down their chins. They turned and fled – BUT in opposite directions, and Tiger pulled so hard that Tapir's tail came off and he was only left with a stump! In great pain he cantered away from both Tiger and the goats, thinking of the drops of blood coming from their mouths.

Tiger ran in the opposite direction thinking how he must untie Tapir's tail from his own. And the goats? They laughed and laughed, and praised the wisdom of Thin Goat who had now saved them three times from terrible danger.

This is an important story for empowering children and young people. The smallest and thinnest goat is the cleverest one, and he looks out for the others. He saves the goats from three types of very frightening dangers: the farmer, the tiger and then the tiger and tapir together: an excellent story for developing coping skills.

Exploration

1. Read through the story together and discuss it, and invite questions.
2. Write the three dangers on the board in large letters so that everyone is clear what they are.
3. Draw a picture of the goats with all the juice dribbling down their chins.
4. Use tiger and goat puppets to tell scenes from the story, with the goats developing very strong voices.
5. Create a group picture of the forest and cut our tigers and goats and put them behind the trees (perhaps adding other animals as well).

Additional Healing Story 3

The Children of Wax: a Story from Africa

Long ago, in Africa, there lived a farming family who grew crops and tended animals. However, they were different from other families because all their children were made of wax. No-one knew why this happened but it was a fact.

The children had to take great care and not go near any fires, and they could not, of course, go outside while the sun was shining. Their father built a special shelter to shield the children from the hot sun and the children rested by day and came out at night. They worked very hard in the fields and tended the animals. Only one of the children yearned for a life beyond the farm and wanted to see the world.

After some time he decided that he would leave his brothers and sisters and take the risk and explore life beyond their shelter. One day, while his siblings were occupied he slipped out of the shelter into the blazing sun. He was only able to go a few steps before the merciless sun melted him and soon he was just a pool of wax.

His brothers and sisters peered out of the door and were very shocked when they saw what had happened. As soon as it became dark they all left the shelter and scooped up the wax that had been their brother. They used the wax to model a wonderful bird and covered it with leaves instead of feathers. Then they placed it on some rocks nearby and went back to the shelter to wait and watch.

When the sun rose in the morning the bird shone in the pink lights of dawn. Then it slowly took off and flew gracefully away into the distance. The children were overjoyed and went to tell their parents what had happened. They knew that their brother would find happiness at last, out there in the world.

Discussion

This is a story about loss and transformation. It is also a story about difference and how it is possible to live with being unconventional. It has elements of adaptation and ends with the triumph of succeeding in a different way.

Exploration

1 Everyone imagines they are candles that are alight, and they slowly melt into puddles of wax.
2 With a partner discuss what it would be like to only come alive at night.
3 Draw and colour the most beautiful bird you can think of.
4 Using clay or play-dough model a bird and think of different things to use as feathers for example, wood-shavings, small twigs, flowers, leaves.
5 In groups of 3 or 4 image your are in the shelter and discuss as a group whether to escape from the hut and discover the big world.
6 Without using words create a scene where one child escapes and the others cannot stop him or her from leaving.

Certificate of Achievement
Awarded to

_____

has shown skills in the following areas:

_____

_____

and has contributed to the group by:

_____

_____

_____   _____
Signed   Date

Warm-Up & Drama Games

These exercises vary from very simple to more complex games. They are ideal as an introduction to 'action learning', and provide a basis for confidence building. A warm-up is just that, it warms up the body and the brain, ready for creative activity. Perhaps their most important function is simply to focus energy. It is important, when choosing warm-ups, that they are linked to the activities in the group and not chosen at random.

I usually start with physical warm-ups, because often there is surplus energy that needs to be focussed and then transformed. My approach does not work with angry expression for its own sake, in the sense of smashing old china or breaking bricks; I use physical energy that expresses angry energy, and then turns it into something more positive.

For example, a physical game of throwing and catching the soft ball focuses scattered energy and allows it to become collaborative energy. A jog around the park enhances the 'feel-good' factor, and prepares group members for focussed group work. In all warm-ups it is important to remember awareness of breathing, whether to create energy or to bring about relaxation.

1   Breathing and voice
(Exercises to be repeated 3 or 4 times.)

1 Breathe in through the nose to a count of 4, and then out through the mouth to a count of 4; keep the shoulders relaxed and the tummy tucked in. Repeat, with a pause for 4 counts between breathing in and out.

2 Take a deep breath in through the nose, and breathe out on the word 'home'.

3 Say 'ho, ho, ho', as loudly as possible. Repeat, increasing volume; and then repeat, becoming quieter.

4 Repeat quickly, 'red leather, yellow leather', 5 times, then 10 times.

5 Repeat quickly, 'a clown with a crown', 5 times, then 10 times.

6 Talk a nonsense language with a partner as fast as possible, and then very slowly as if feeling sleepy.

2 Strong movement

1 Invite the group to scatter around the room and call out 'freeze!'; everyone stands absolutely still. Then call out, 'go!'; everyone moves again. Repeat several times until unison is achieved.

2 Suggest contrasting movements, such as running around in a circle and scattering all over the place.

3 Move around the room as if being blown.

4 Run around and jump very high.

5 Stand absolutely still and create a silence.

3 Rhythm and drum work

1 Invite the group to sit in a circle and clap a simple rhythm until they are clapping in unison.

2 Divide the group in half: one half clapping at the original speed, the other twice as fast.

3 Play with the idea of different rhythms; invite the group to make suggestions.

4 Allow group members to use a drum and lead the rhythm; the person with the drum leads and the group copies.

5 Use a drumming CD, and suggest that everyone copies a rhythm.

4 More rhythm and drum work

1 Using a drumbeat, suggest everyone walks to the beat.

2 Try marching to the drumbeat, first on the spot, and then around the room

3 March with a partner and synchronise the movements.

4 March with three people and create the marching 'wheel', in which the person at the centre of the wheel marches on the spot, while the others move around in a circle. (Quite a challenge!)

5 Attempt to march backwards, staying in the wheel. (A big challenge!)

5 Physical work

1. Throw the soft ball between group members, while running around the room; vary between throwing the ball randomly, and shouting the name of the person who should catch it.
2. Hold hands in a circle and pull each way, keeping the circle intact.
3. Hold hands in a circle, and then move over and under everyone until a tight knot is formed. Slowly undo the knot without letting go of the hands.
4. Pass a clap or a rhythm around the circle to create a ripple effect, as if the sound is continuous.
5. Stand in a circle; each person sits down one at a time, but if two go down at the same time, everyone has to start from the beginning. Repeat the exercise, this time standing up from sitting.

6 Synchronised games

1. Everyone stands in a large circle; each person takes one step forward, but if two people move at the same time, the game starts again.
2. Repeat the exercise, this time moving out of the circle, one step at a time.
3. Everyone stands in a large circle and counts, 'one, two, three, four'. On 'four' each person looks at someone else; if the same person is also looking at them, they change places. Keep repeating until there has been plenty of movement across the group.
4. Variation: number everyone in the group (just go around the circle and have each person say their number); call out two numbers and those people have to change places.
5. More difficult: call out two sets of numbers, such as '2 and 7' and '4 and 8'. Those four people change places, with everyone taking care not to bump into the others as they cross the circle.

7 Clapping and rhythm

1. Pass a single clap around the circle, one person following the next and keeping up the rhythm.
2. Repeat in the opposite direction, varying the pace if group is ready.
3. Change to a double clap and send it around in one direction.
4. Vary the pace and send in the opposite direction
5. Change to a triple clap and send it in one direction; at the same time send a double clap in the opposite direction.

8 Rhythm in words and music

1. Share the idea that certain jobs have their own rhythmic chant, so that everyone works together, for example: pulling a rope, rowing a boat.

2. Invite everyone to sit in the circle and teach the chant: 'Aayee oh, aayee oh, ay, ay, ay, ay, aayee oh.' Practise until synchronised.

3. Add the movement of rowing a boat to the rhythm; practise until the chant and movement are synchronised.

4. Explain to the group that words used together in a sentence have a rhythm. Invite members to think of famous, rhythmic catchphrases, such as: 'It's goodnight from him – and goodnight from me'; or 'Nice to see you – to see you nice'.

5. Ask the group to think about the rhythms in music and song lyrics. Invite group members to think of music they like with a strong rhythm and words, and practise it together.

9 Rhyming words and rhythmic words

(Use one of the rhyming dictionaries suggested in Resources, 'Useful Reading'.)

1. Invite the group to sit in the circle and clap, while saying words that rhyme, for example: 'splat, mat, cat, rat'; or 'hi, my, try, cry, fry'.

2. Share words that have a strong rhythm, such as: 'dinner, dinner, dinner'; or 'hokey, cokey, cokey, cokey'.

3. Invite everyone to make up two lines that rhyme, for example: 'I went to school, and broke a rule'; or 'I went to school, and fell in a pool.' Encourage more and more nonsense, such as: 'I went to school, riding a mule.'

4. In pairs, write down (or just say) as many words as possible that rhyme with 'song' (one rhyming dictionary lists 21). Then add slight pronunciation variations, for example, 'tongue'.

5. Give group members working in pairs a first line, such as: 'Today I am going to cook a song.' Each pair adds three more lines.

10 Drama and focus games

1. 'Varoom': With everyone standing in a circle, one person calls 'Varoom', and looks at someone else. That person says 'Varoom' to another, and so on. There's no 'varooming' someone next to you, and no repetition back and forth to same person.

2. 'Varoom Plus': 'Varoom' someone in the group, who then chooses to call 'Bazooka', and to hold both their arms in front of them, hands clasped, pointing towards someone on the opposite side of group. Or they can call out 'Varoom Plus', at which everyone crosses their arms on their chest. The leader starts 'Varoom Plus' again

3 Variation: As above, but adding a third action and sound: 'Lalala'. If someone shouts 'Lalala', everyone has to put their hands over their ears and shout, 'Lalala' four times!

4 Invite members of the group to add an action with a nonsense word, but ask them to avoid movements that could involve hitting other people; try to keep all extended movement in front, rather than to the side, of the body.

5 Invite members of the group to choose one of the games to practise very quickly.

11   More drama and focus games

1 'Bees Knees': Everyone runs around the room with one hand on one knee, calling out 'Bees Knees'. Each person has to touch four pairs of knees; then retrace steps and find and touch the knees touched the first time.

2 'Aliens': Everyone stands in a circle. The leader is in the middle and turns around slowly, then points with clasped hands towards one person, calling 'Medan'. The person who has been pointed at is an 'alien' and has to duck down on one knee. The two people on either side of the 'alien' face each other and call out 'Nimro'. The 'alien' between them (still ducking) calls back 'Feelib', and can then stand up again. *However*, if anyone says the wrong word, they have to stay on one knee or crouch down on one knee if they are still standing. Repeat until everyone (except, of course, the leader) is an 'alien' and is sitting on the floor because they have made three mistakes (crouching on one knee for the first mistake, both knees for the second, finally sitting on the floor for the third).

3 'Slapping Hands': Kneel in a circle and place the left hand, palm down, in front of you; place your right hand to right of the next person's left hand, so that everyone's hands are crossing the hands of the people next to them, all around circle. Send a slap around the circle to the right, from left hand to left hand! Repeat, still sending the slap to the right, but this time from right hand to right hand. Then try sending the slaps in the opposite direction, to the left. (This warm-up requires patience and skill!).

12   Rhyming and nonsense play

1 'I did not go to school, because ...' Everyone thinks of the silliest reason, such as: 'I met a bulldozer on the way'; 'it was raining ice cream'; or 'it was Sunday anyway'.

2 'We cannot play football, because ...' Possible endings: 'they have planted potatoes on the pitch'; 'the guinea pig ate the football'; or 'they are playing hockey instead'.

3 In pairs, one person mimes a job and the other asks, 'What are you doing?' The answer should not fit the mime, for example: the person miming is pretending to dig the garden, but they answer 'fixing the bike', 'mixing a cake', or 'blowing my nose'.

4 As above, but when the person 'digging' the garden gives their answer, their partner starts to mime what they have said. Using the example above, they might start to blow their nose.

5 As above, but the person who was 'digging' the garden responds by saying, 'Why are you going to sleep? I said I was blowing my nose.' Then they start a different nonsense dialogue, such as beginning with a mime of feeding the birds.

13 Games for improvisation

1 Run a three-legged race with a partner, without tying the ankles.

2 Create 'stepping stones' with pieces of newspaper. Everyone has to cross the 'river' or the 'chasm' beneath the 'stones' without tearing the paper. Elaborate by having two people moving from 'stone to stone' together.

3 The group pretend they are medical students, and someone comes to give them a talk on knitting.

4 The group pretend they are housewives and househusbands, and someone comes to give them a talk on brain surgery.

5 Two people are fruit and vegetable stallholders, and call out what they are selling and for what price; they try to compete with each other.

6 In pairs, one partner is a customer and the other is trying to show off all the best points of a car without knowing anything about them; the 'car salesman' has to bluff their way through.

7 In pairs, one person is a student and the other a physics teacher; in reality the 'physics teacher' is a piano teacher and knows nothing about physics.

8 In small groups, one person leads the others across different types of terrain, such as desert, rainforest, ice flow, stream, farmyard, and so on. The group members don't know what the terrain is, so they follow and then guess at the end.

9 Repeat, but this time the groups are on ice that is about to crack, or in a place where they can see that there will shortly be a landslide; tell the groups everyone has to move quickly and lightly.

All of these exercises can be developed into situations or stories. Many will become favourites to be repeated. Very importantly, group members will start to develop their own versions of the exercises.

References & Further Reading

Bowlby J. (1988) *A Secure Base: Clinical Application of Attachment Theory*, Routledge, London.

Campbell J. (1993) *The Hero with a Thousand Faces*, Bollingen, Princeton.

Creative Care (2012) 'Creating an alternative pathway'(booklet), Rowan Tree Trust, Somerset.

Erikson E. (1951/1995) *Childhood and Society*, Vintage, London.

Gerhardt C. (2004) *Why Love Matters: How Affection Shapes a Baby's Brain*, Bruner-Routledge, Hove.

Hickson A. (2011) *How to Stop Bullying: 101 Strategies that Really Work*, Speechmark, Milton Keynes.

Jennings S. (2004) *Creative Storytelling with Children at Risk*, Speechmark, Milton Keynes.

Jennings S. (2011) *Healthy Attachments and Neuro-Dramatic-Play*, Jessica Kingsley Publishers, London.

Jennings S. (2012) *The Anger Management Toolkit: Understanding & Transforming Anger in Children & Young People*, Hinton House, Buckingham.

Jennings S. (2013) *101 Ideas for Managing Challenging Behaviour*, Hinton House, Buckingham.

Jennings S. (2014) 'Applying an Embodiment-Projection-Role framework in groupwork with children', in *Play Therapy Today*, Prendiville E. (ed.), Routledge, London.

Lahad M. (2013) *The "BASIC Ph" Model of Coping and Resiliency: Theory, Research and Cross-Cultural Application*, Jessica Kingsley Publishers, London.

Lahad M. (2000) *Creative Supervision*, Jessica Kingsley Publishers, London.

McCall Smith, A. (1989) *Children of Wax: African Folk Tales*, Interlink Books, New York.

McCarthy D. (2007) *If You Turned into a Monster*, Jessica Kingsley Publishers, London.

McCarthy D. (2012) *A Manual of Dynamic Play Therapy: Helping Things Fall Apart, the Paradox of Play*, Jessica Kingsley Publishers, London.

Pearson, J., Smail, M. & Watts, P. (2013) *Dramatherapy with Myth and Fairytale: The Golden Stories of Sesame*, Jessica Kingsley Publishers, London.

Rutter M. (1997) *Psychosocial Disturbances in Young People: Challenges for Prevention*, Cambridge University Press, Cambridge.

Schrader C. (2012) *Ritual Theatre: the Power of Dramatic Ritual in Personal Development Groups and Clinical Practice*, Jessica Kingsley Publishers, London.

Sunderland M. (2006) *What Every Parent Needs to Know*, D.K. Publishing, London.

Whitehead, C. (2001) 'Social Mirrors and Shared Experiential Worlds', *Journal of Consciousness Studies* Vol. 8(4): 12–32.

Information on Training

Training is available in the UK, Romania, Malaysia and Czech Republic.

Training in Neuro-Dramatic-Play, EPR and Trauma is divided into three developmental stages:

1. Creative Care: attachment and nature-nurture; sensory and echo-play, rhythmic and ritual play; breathing, sound, voice and movement; sand play, dramatic play, monsters.
2. Therapeutic Ritual & Storytelling: non-verbal creativity; structured stories and rituals; therapeutic storytelling and creative visualisation, Six Part Story Assessment, puppets, Hero's Journey. rites of passage.
3. Theatre of Resilience: sensory and bodywork, 'mandalas', role-play and dramatisation; culture-based performance and interactive stories; celebrations and ceremonies, body-mind-spirit integration.

NDP is demonstrated and explained in the following titles:

Jennings S. (2011) *Healthy Attachments and Neuro-Dramatic-Play*, Jessica Kingsley Publishers, London.

Jennings S. (2012) *The Neuro-Dramatic-Play, Play-Book, Part 1*, Healing Tree.

DVD: *Neuro-Dramatic-Play: Journey to Playfulness and Creativity*, Healing Tree.

101 Activities & Ideas

* Creative and practical solutions to issues around emotional well-being in young people. Many teachers, care workers and therapists are challenged by difficult behaviours, and families often feel lost for solutions to sudden outbursts or young people's feelings of alienation and lack of self-esteem.
* Containing a host of ideas for home, school and youth groups, the books will help to tackle these difficult issues in a positive and active way. There are no magic answers, but the ideas aim to empower young people to find solutions to some of their own difficulties, while providing guidance for more positive directions.
* The books adopt a 'hands-on' approach with a firm and enabling attitude and provide a sound practical basis for active intervention for behaviour change.

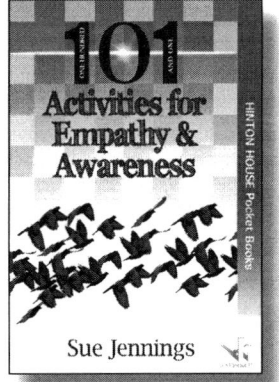

101 Activities for Empathy & Awareness
ISBN: 978-1-906531-33-1

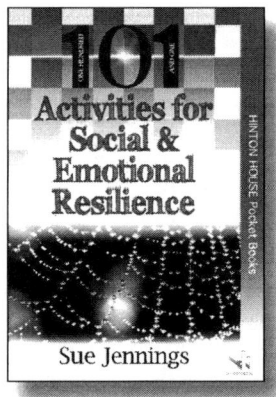

101 Activities for Social & Emotional Resilience
ISBN: 978-1-906531-46-1

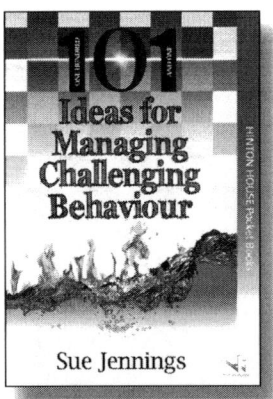

101 Ideas for Managing Challenging Behaviour
ISBN: 978-1-906531-44-7

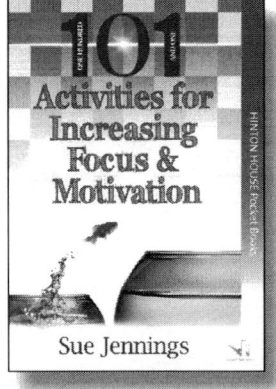

101 Activities for Increasing Focus & Motivation
ISBN: 978-1-906531-45-4

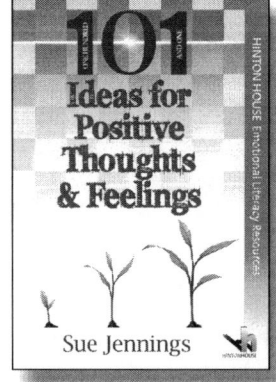

101 Ideas for Positive Thoughts & Feelings
ISBN: 978-1-906531-47-8

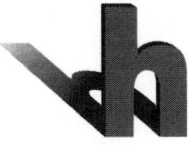

www.hintonpublishers.com